TELECOURSE STUDY GUIDE
FOR

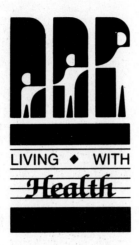

LIVING ◆ WITH

Health

TELECOURSE STUDY GUIDE
FOR

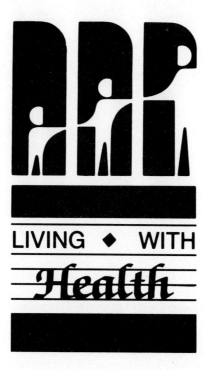

LIVING ◆ WITH

Health

DONNA BECK RICHARDS, R.N., M.S.

Dallas County Community College District

In cooperation with McGraw-Hill, Inc.

New York   St. Louis   San Francisco   Auckland   Bogotá   Caracas

Lisbon   London   Madrid   Mexico City   Milan   Montreal   New Delhi

San Juan   Singapore   Sydney   Tokyo   Toronto

TELECOURSE STUDY GUIDE FOR LIVING WITH HEALTH

This book is printed on acid-free paper.

3 4 5 6 7 8 9 0   AGM   AGM   9 0 9 8 7 6 5 4

ISBN 0-07-015187-3

The editor was Sylvia Shepard;
the production supervisor was Elizabeth Strange.
Arcata Graphics/Martinsburg was printer and binder.

Richard Bach, *Jonathan Livingston Seagull*, New York, Macmillan, 1990.
Rahima Baldwin and Terra Palmarini, *Pregnant Feelings*, Berkeley, Calif., Celestial Arts, 1986.
Norman Cousins, *Anatomy of an Illness as Perceived by the Patient: Reflections on Healing and Regeneration*,
New York, Bantam, 1981.
Larry Dossey, M.D., *Beyond Illness*, New York, Random House, 1985.
Robert A. Johnson, *We*, San Francisco, Harper, 1985.
Elisabeth Kübler-Ross, M.D., *On Life after Death*, Berkeley, Calif., Celestial Arts Publisher, 1991.
Anne Morrow Lindbergh, *Gift from the Sea*, New York, Pantheon Books, 1975.

For

Jim

Barbara, Karen

Ethel

In Memory Of

Gordon and Bobby

Without the high and the low, the hot and the cold, life would be a seamless, undifferentiated experience of sameness. Without the rhythms of health and illness and birth and death, we would fall heir not to a state of pristine perfection, but to one of experiential anesthesia. Our health strategy must always be supplemented with this awareness. For if we ever achieved our goal of total health, we would find, not fulfillment, but emptiness. Health, if seen as wholeness, guards against this dreadful error, for the whole contains all—even, we must all recall, the opposites of birth and death, pain and pleasure, illness and health.

Larry Dossey, M.D.
Beyond Illness

Table of Contents

To the Student

Welcome to **Living With Health**! You and I are about to take a long journey. We will travel over 30,000 miles, meet some of the nation's top experts in the fields of medicine and health, and share the lives of dozens of special people. If I just described these people to you, you might wonder why I define them as "special," because they are much like you and I — just "folks" living their lives, coping with the ups and downs that life has to offer. You will find as you meet them, that indeed they are special, as are you and I. Each of us is unique, yet we all share some of the same ups and downs, hopes and fears, pain and celebration.

As we travel and visit with these people, we will see their lifestyles, hear about their experiences, and understand what it takes to achieve and maintain a high quality of health and well-being. Throughout our travels in this course, we will be looking at health in its five dimensions: physical, emotional, intellectual, social, and spiritual. All these aspects of our being come together to make us a whole, healthy person. (Not everyone includes the last, spiritual, in their list, but I have a feeling that, when you see it in the context of this course, you will certainly include it in your life.) In our time together, we will discuss the topics related to health within this framework of the dimensions of health. We will discover that health is a dynamic process rather than a static point. We will find that most of our good health is within our control and is our responsibility to maintain.

The fifteen months that I have committed to the development of **Living With Health** have been life changing for me. I hope the months that we spend together will change yours as well. The purpose of **Living With Health** is to give you tools to make lifestyle choices and decisions that will improve the quality of your health and well-being. Whether you choose to use them to shape your own life will, of course, be your decision. I very much hope you will find these tools useful to your life.

Donna Beck Richards

Course Organization

Living With Health is designed as a comprehensive learning package consisting of three elements: Study Guide, Textbook, and Video Programs.

Study Guide

This Study Guide acts as your daily instructor. Each lesson begins with a brief essay, which provides you with an **Overview** and a context for the material presented in that lesson. Following this Overview the **Learning Objectives** inform you of specific objectives. Next the **Study Assignment** directs you to the text and video assignments. **Text Focus Points** keyed to the reading material are intended to help you get the most from your reading. A listing of the **Experts Interviewed** for each lesson and the **Video Focus Points** will help you learn from the video presentation. The **Individual Health Plan** helps you apply what you have learned to your own health. **Enrichment Opportunities** encourage you to go beyond the elements required in the course. Finally, a **Practice Test** allows you to sample the types of questions you will encounter on exams.

If you follow the Study Guide recommendations for each lesson carefully, you should successfully accomplish all of the requirements for this course.

Textbook

In addition to the Study Guide, there is a textbook required for this course:

> *Life and Health: Targeting Wellness,* 1st Edition, by Levy, Dignan, and Shirreffs, McGraw-Hill, Inc., 1992

This textbook examines health and wellness as a balance of the five dimensions: physical, emotional, intellectual, social, and spiritual. These concepts form the basis for the presentation of the major issues and topics in health today.

Video Programs

Each video program is correlated with the Study Guide and the Text assigment for that lesson. Be sure to read the Video Focus Points in the Study Guide before you watch the program. The video programs are presented in a documentary format and are designed to bring analysis and application to the issues being disussed. Watch them closely. If the programs are broadcast more than once in your area, or if video tapes are available at your college, you might find it helpful to watch the video programs more than once.

How to Use The Study Guide

As in anything you do in your life, the information you will get from this course will be related to the work you put into it. I do not promise this will always be easy. You have probably been introduced to many of the concepts already. This course is different in that you will be invited to actually apply the principles you are studying to your own life as you are studying them.

The following is the format for each study guide lesson with suggestions on how to use each part.

Study Guide Lesson

Quote

These are simply some "words of wisdom" that I found relevant and chose to share with you. I hope you enjoy them and that they cause you to stop for a moment and think about what they are saying.

Overview

This section is a brief summary of what the lesson will cover. In some instances, there is information not in the text or other comments I think you should know about. Read this before doing any of the rest of the lesson.

Learning Objectives

The primary lesson goal and objectives related to this goal are included in this section. These reflect the overall knowledge that you will be responsible for.

Study Assignments

> **Textbook** — This is the reading assignment critical to the lesson. You must complete the textbook assignment. I recommend that you do this before viewing the video portion.

> **Video** — This is the video that supports this lesson. This is integral to the lesson. It and the textbook are both required assignments.

Key Terms

These are important terms, many of which will be new to you. You are responsible for understanding what they mean.

Text Focus Points

The Text Focus Points guide your reading in the text. You should read the text focus points before you read your textbook. You are responsible for the information in the textbook covered by the text focus points. It is a good idea to write out or at least take notes about each focus point after you study your textbook.

Experts Interviewed

Listed here are the experts interviewed in the video program. The list includes their affiliation for your information.

Video Focus Points

The Video Focus Points guide your viewing of the video program. You should study the video focus points before watching the program because you will be responsible for the information covered by the video focus points. It is a good idea to write out the answer to each focus point after you view the program.

Individual Health Plan

The assignment in this section should be completed in your journal at the time you do the rest of the lesson. You should plan on turning in portions of your journal as required by your instructor, so it is recommended that you keep a loose leaf notebook for your journal.

Enrichment Opportunities

These exercises are designed to guide you if you want or need further information on the lesson or if your instructor requires them to be done.

Practice Test

These questions are similar to those which will be included in the objective portion of your tests. You should complete this after every lesson. Check your answers in the answer key and review the text or video program for any questions you missed. The essay questions on your test will be similar to the focus points and objectives. You will be expected to apply information you have learned to answer the essay questions.

Answer Key

The answers to the Practice Test questions are listed here. Page, Text Focus Point, Video Focus Point, and Objective references are also listed.

Study Guidelines

The quickest and most efficient way for you to cover the important points in each lesson is to follow these study guidelines. For each lesson:

1. Read the **Overview**, **Learning Objectives**, **Key Terms** and **Text Focus Points** for the lesson.
2. Complete the **Study Assignment**, keeping the **Key Terms** and **Text Focus Points** in mind.
3. Write your responses to the **Text Focus Points**, going back to the text if you are not certain you know the answers.
4. Note the names of the major **Experts Interviewed**, then examine the **Video Focus Points**.
5. View the video program with the **Key Terms** and **Video Focus Points** in mind. Take only brief notes while viewing.
6. Immediately after viewing the video program, write detailed responses to the **Video Focus Points**, referring to your notes to help you.
7. Define each **Key Term**.
8. Take the **Practice Test** to check your understanding of the concepts presented in the lesson.
9. Compare your answers to the **Answer Key** located at the end of the lesson. If you answered incorrectly, the key provides references so that you can review the material from which each question was taken.
10. Apply your learning through the completion of your **Individual Health Plan**. Extend your knowledge by acting on one or more of the suggested **Enrichment Opportunities**.

Acknowledgements

No project such as this is ever the work of one person. Many people shared the commitment to **Living With Health** and I thank each of them.

To Paul Bosner, Director of Production, who also functioned as one of the producers, I owe thanks for an incredible experience, for keeping us on track, and for sharing a lifetime of experience with this neophyte. Thanks to Mark Birnbaum, Producer/Director, for his creativity and sensitivity to the subject matter and putting up with the content specialist. To Nora Coto Busby, Instructional Designer, I owe the instructional quality of this course, and thanks for being a real friend who kept me centered throughout. Karen C. Austen, Researcher, did well-focused research, too many other duties to mention, and asked questions that made us all think. David Molina, Associate Producer, kept us all organized and on the road, and had the answer to any question we could ever think of.

Without the work of Darise Error and Michelle Miller, Production Assistants, there would have been no video programs. I thank Letitia Richardson and Lannie Waggy for all those details that added to the project. My admiration goes to Janet Fulton, Vicki Metz, and Michael Coleman for their talented editing of the video and to the camera and audio experts who brought the whole thing to life. Other special people to this project were Pamela K. Quinn, Vice President of the R. Jan LeCroy Center for Educational Telecommunications, and all the staff at the Center who were so involved. Thanks also to Margot Olson, Test Design Specialist, and Nancy Ward of the Word Works. Appreciation to all those on the advisory committees who shared their wisdom to improve my efforts.

Finally, thanks to all those special people who shared their lives with us, and all you students who taught me so much through the years.

Donna Beck Richards

Living with Health telecourse is produced by the Dallas County Community College District, R. Jan LeCroy Center for Educational Telecommunications, in association with Northern Illinois Learning Resources Cooperative, Northern California Telecommunications Consortium and in cooperation with McGraw-Hill, Inc. Publishing Company.

TELECOURSE STUDY GUIDE
FOR

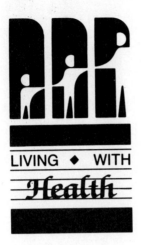

LIVING ◆ WITH

Health

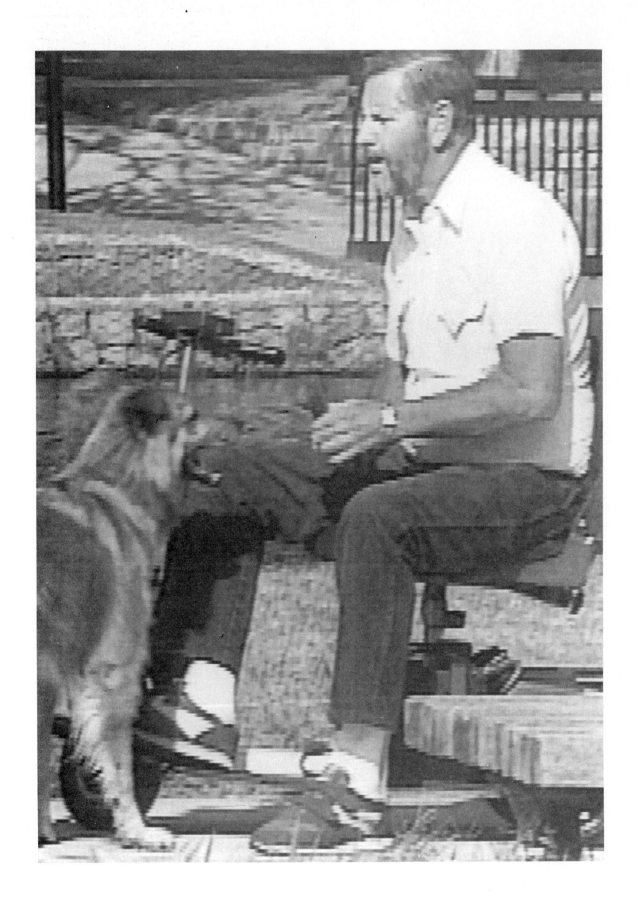

Lesson 1

Invitation to Health

If you can force your heart and nerve and sinew
To serve your turn long after they are gone,
And so hold on when there is nothing in you
Except the Will which says to them: "Hold on"

Rudyard Kipling

Overview

How do you define health? If you are thinking merely in terms of getting enough exercise and eating the "right" foods, you are missing four-fifths of the ingredients of health. If you define health as the absence of disease, you are missing even more.

Follow us into a much more exciting and interesting world of health and wellness. Think of five dimensions that define our health — physical, emotional, intellectual, spiritual, and social. Each of these interact and interrelate to form who and what we are. Each has a major impact on our well-being. If all are not nurtured and maintained, we will be less than whole. A significant part of our being will be needy. In each of us, one or another of these dimensions may be more or less developed, but they are there.

To add to the complexity and wonder of all this, our lifestyle and its components are the most important influences on these dimensions of health. So how we live our lives has more to do with our health than any other component. Before we talk more about the components of lifestyle today, think for a moment about how our lifestyles have changed through the generations. Our lifestyle has evolved from that of hunting and gathering food to one of sedentary work and fast food establishments. At the same time, strides in medicine and technology have conquered many of the diseases that killed our ancestors. Until recently, our health was considered more a matter of luck than individual responsibility.

Many bacterial and viral diseases have been conquered that were out of our own control to prevent. We now realize that the killer diseases of today frequently are related intimately to lifestyle. In other words, our lifestyle may be killing us. If the idea of killing yourself is startling, let's talk more about what we mean by the lifestyles that have such positive and negative influence on our health.

Our lifestyle means the way we spend the major parts of our lives: working, communicating, recreating, relating, consuming, etc. How we design and structure these components determines, to a large degree, how healthy we are. Though we cannot change our heredity, we do have the power to make the lifestyle decisions that will improve the quality of our health.

Making these decisions, setting our goals, assessing our health status, and then actually carrying out our plan is not always easy. We have to constantly evaluate our progress, sometimes adjust our goals, and just "keep on trucking." The outcome is definitely worth the effort, for there is no doubt that we will improve the quality of our lives — **and have lots of fun while we are doing it!**

Learning Objectives

Goal: You should be able to explain the five dimensions of health, the impact of lifestyle on health, and the importance of health goals.

Objectives: Upon completion of this lesson, you should be able to:

1. Define health in terms of the integration and balance of the five dimensions of health.

2. Describe the ways in which heredity, lifestyle components, and self-efficacy affect our health today, and in the future.

3. Analyze the process of establishing health priorities and personal health goals.

Study Assignments

Pay careful attention to the following assignments. The chapter number may not be the same as the lesson number.

Textbook: Chapter 1, "The Concept of Health," pp. 2-27

Video: "Invitation to Health"

Key Terms

Watch for these terms and pay particular attention to what each one means, as you follow the textbook and video.

Hardiness	**Genes**
Homeostasis	**Lifestyle**
Regeneration	**Self-efficacy**

Textbook Focus Points

Before you read the textbook assignment, review the following points to help focus your thoughts. After you complete the assignment, write out your responses to reinforce what you have learned.

1. Define health in terms of the five distinct, but interrelated dimensions.

2. Explain the five dimensions of health, and the role they play in an individual's health.

3. Explain the integration of health in terms of health and balance.

4. Discuss the role of heredity and lifestyle in maintaining health.

5. How do the various lifestyle components influence the dimensions of health?

6. What is self-efficacy, and what role does it play in maintaining one's health?

---

7. How are individual's needs and wants important in the process of setting health goals?

8. Analyze the process of personal health goal setting, and discuss the importance of each aspect.

9. List and explain the steps an individual must complete in the self assessment process of setting health goals.

Expert Interviewed

In the video segment of this lesson, the following health professional shares his expertise to help you understand the material presented.

Steven N. Blair, P.E.D., Director of Epidemiology, Cooper Institute for Aerobics Research, Dallas, Texas

Video Focus Points

The following questions are designed to help you get the most from the video segment of this lesson. Review them before you watch the video. After viewing the video segment, write responses to reinforce what you have learned.

1. How are definitions of health and wellness different today than in the past?

2. Why is it important that the five dimensions, physical, emotional, intellectual, social, and spiritual be balanced in one's life?

3. Explain the importance of lifestyle decisions on one's health and the balance of the five dimensions. Include differences from person-to-person and from time-to-time.

Individual Health Plan

This portion of the lesson is designed to enable you to apply the information you have learned to your own life situation and improve the quality of your life. You should do any exercise assigned, complete the journal portion of the plan, then put this portion of the health plan into practice in your life.

Using the self assessment, "Is Your Lifestyle Good for Your Health," on page 11 of your textbook, evaluate your present health lifestyle. Use this information and the self-assessment steps in the textbook, pages 21-24, to begin your journal writing. In your journal, develop an in-depth assessment of the status of your health, lifestyle and choices. Begin to set your health and wellness goals with this exercise.

Enrichment Opportunities

These suggestions guide you if you want more information on this lesson, want to explore new ideas, or if your instructor requires it. If you are doing this section as a course requirement, consult with your instructor for specific guidelines or directions.

1. Conduct interviews with some of your friends and family. Evaluate their lifestyle choices, based on what you have learned from this lesson.

2. If you smoke, **stop!** (Additional information in Lesson 19.)

3. After consulting with your instructor and possibly your physician, begin an exercise program. (Additional information in Lesson 5.)

Practice Test

After reading the assignment and watching the video, you should be able to answer the Practice Test questions. Tests also include essay questions that are similar to the Text Focus Points, the Video Focus Points, and the Objectives. When you have completed the Practice Test questions, turn to the Answer Key to score your answers..

1. Which of the following statements best describes the modern view of health?
   A. Health refers to the ability to cope with emotional problems.
   B. Health has many aspects, each of which contributes to well-being.
   C. Health is predominantly controlled by heredity and environment.
   D. Health largely depends on maintaining body functions.

2. In order to achieve homeostasis, the body seeks to maintain a balance between factors such as temperature, blood pressure, and
   A. genes.
   B. lifestyle.
   C. weight.
   D. heart rate.

3. Which of the following statements is true of lifestyle?
   A. Lifestyle implies a pattern of behavior rather than an isolated event.
   B. All components of lifestyle are under an individual's control.
   C. Individuals generally make lifestyle choices only after evaluating alternatives.
   D. Lifestyle is related primarily to emotional health.

4. Financial setbacks, disagreements with friends, and accidents are examples of stressful situations that test an individual's
   A. working style.
   B. consuming style.
   C. coping style.
   D. relating style.

5. Confidence in ability to plan and control one's own behaviors and lifestyle components is referred to as
   A. coping style.
   B. self-efficacy.
   C. emotional health.
   D. hardiness.

6. According to Abraham Maslow's theories, which of the following is an example of a higher-level need?
   A. Safety
   B. Shelter
   C. Self-sufficiency
   D. Love

7. An important benefit of setting goals is the opportunity to
   A. experience failure.
   B. measure progress.
   C. eliminate trade-offs.
   D. control hereditary factors.

8. Health is defined as
   A. being free of disease.
   B. feeling happy.
   C. functioning at a high level.
   D. staying alive.

9. When the five dimensions of health are out of balance, the individual is most likely to feel
   A. disease free.
   B. ill at ease.
   C. stress free.
   D. in control.

10. Most major health problems of today are attributed to
    A. infection.
    B. lifestyle.
    C. immune system problems.
    D. viruses.

11. The possession of an optimistic and committed approach to life is known as _____.

---

12. A person's overall way of living is called _____.

13. As you conduct an ongoing self-assessment in achieving goals, it is important to regularly evaluate your _____.

14. Quality of life, resulting in a high level of functioning in all aspects of living, is a definition for _____.

15. One of the major keys to good health is our choice of _____.

True or False

16. It is important that dimensions of health be well integrated into lifestyle.

17. Communication style is simply the way we speak to people.

18. Though Americans seem to have begun to take a more active role in the pursuit of health and well-being, they don't practice more safety measures.

19. Wellness is a generic term that refers to a healthful approach to living.

20. One can live a very healthy life even if one or two of the dimensions are out of balance.

Answer Key

These are the correct answers with reference to the Learning Objectives, and to the source of the information: the Textbook Focus Points, Levy, *et al. Life and Health*, and the Video Focus Points. Page numbers are also given for the Textbook Focus Points. "KT" indicates questions with Key Terms defined.

Question	Answer	Learning Objective	Textbook Focus Point (page no.)		Video Focus Point
1.	B	1.1	1 (p. 5)		
2.	D	1.1	3 (p. 9)	KT	
3.	A	1.2	4 (pp. 12-13)	KT	
4.	C	1.2	5 (p. 14)		
5.	B	1.2	6 (p. 17)	KT	
6.	C	1.3	7 (p. 19)		
7.	B	1.3	8 (p. 19)		
8.	C	1.1			1
9.	B	1.1			2
10.	B	1.2			3
11.	hardiness	1.1	2 (p. 5)		
12.	lifestyle	1.2	4 (p. 12)	KT	
13.	progress	1.3	9 (p. 24)		
14.	health	1.1			1
15.	lifestyle	1.2			3
16.	T	1.1	1 (p. 9)		
17.	F	1.2	5 (p. 14)		
18.	F	1.2	10 (p. 24)		
19.	T	1.1			1
20.	F	1.1			2

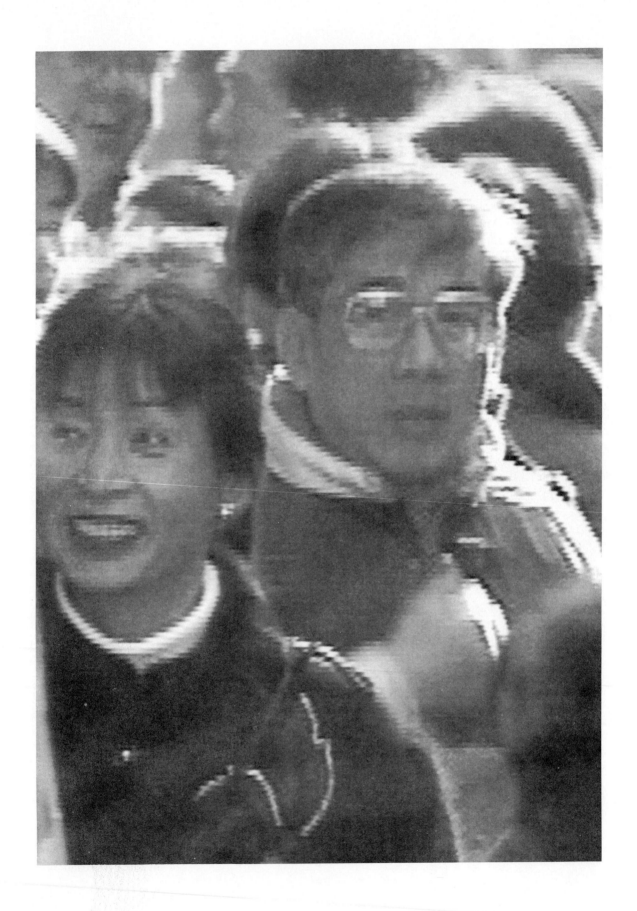

Lesson 2

Stress

Dig the well before you are thirsty.

Chinese proverb

Overview

When asked whether stress is good or bad, most of us will say **bad** without hesitation. The fact is — if you do not have stress in your life, you are **dead**! Stress actually keeps us alive! In reality stress is neither good nor bad, yet it is both good and bad. Now are you thoroughly confused? The way in which we cope with stress is the factor that makes each stress a positive or negative factor in our lives.

We all encounter stress everyday in our lives, some tiny and routine, some large, unavoidable, and terrifying, and some very intense and personal in our relationships with others. Our ability to understand the nature of stress, our physiological and psychological responses to stress, and how we manage and reduce the negative effects of stress have major impact on our health and well-being.

No matter what the stress is, if we perceive a threat, our bodies have certain physical ways of responding. Increased heart rate, rapid breathing, elevated blood pressure, increased mental alertness are all part of a three-stage process, defined by Dr. Hans Selye, as the general adaptation syndrome (GAS). The brain, autonomic nervous system, and endocrine system are all involved in our complex physiological response to stress.

Our personality also has a great deal to do with how well we cope with stress. If we believe in ourselves and our abilities, view stress as a normal part of life, and look at life changes in a positive way, we will be far more likely to cope effectively with the stress in our lives.

Stress, however, can have a very negative effect on our behavior and our ability to resist or withstand various diseases. If we are not coping with stress effectively, we may turn to drugs, alcohol, or tobacco instead of dealing with the stress. We may also become depressed, lack concentration, and even engage in acts that increase our risk of injury. Stress has also been linked to an increased risk of certain diseases such as hypertension, heart disease, diabetes, peptic ulcers, mental disorders, and others. Burnout and other job related stress can also present major problems in our lives.

Stress is an inevitable part of our lives, and in fact can be a very positive force in our health. Our goal should not be to remove stress from our lives, but to manage it and reduce its negative effects. We can use stress to motivate us to achieve a higher quality of life.

Simple "band-aid" stress management techniques, such as taking a break from working or studying, surprisingly can offer immediate relief. More complex techniques, such as progressive relaxation, meditation, and autogenic training, are relatively easy to learn and can make a real difference in our lives. In addition to these, learning to approach our lives and stressors in different ways, managing our time effectively, practicing general good health measures, and believing in ourselves and our abilities will give us the tools we need to manage our stress in a healthy way.

Learning Objectives

Goal: You should be able to explain stress, its physiological and psychological effects, the impact of stress on the individual, and the most common stress management techniques.

Objectives: Upon completion of this lesson, you should be able to:

1. Explain the importance of stress, the sources and types of stress, and how people respond to stress.

2. Restate the physiological and psychological effects of stress, including the General Adaption Syndrome, and the role of personality.

3. Comment on the impact of stress on behavior and on the various diseases, including the economic and social costs of stress.

4. Describe several techniques useful in managing stress and some behaviors effective in avoiding or reducing stress.

Study Assignments

Pay careful attention to the following assignments. The chapter number may not be the same as the lesson number.

Textbook Chapter 2, "Stress and Its Management," pp. 28-52

Video: "Stress"

Key Terms

Watch for these terms and pay particular attention to what each one means, as you follow the textbook and video.

Stress	Type A personality/behavior
Stressor	Type B personality/behavior
Eustress	Progressive relaxation
Distress	Autogenic training
General adaption syndrome (GAS)	Biofeedback
Endocrine system	Cognitive appraisal
Hormones	

Textbook Focus Points

Before you read the textbook assignment, review the following points to help focus your thoughts. After you complete the assignment, write out your responses to reinforce what you have learned.

1. State the importance of stress in our lives, and how different people respond to stress.

2. Describe the sources of stress. Include types of stress, situational stressors, and differentiate between acute and chronic stress.

3. Distinguish between "bad" stress and "good" stress and between the effects of major life events and everyday stressors on health.

4. Explain the General Adaptation Syndrome (GAS) and the contributions of Hans Selye and Richard Lazarus to health research.

5. Describe the physiological effects of the stress mechanism on the body.

6. What role does personality play in responding to stress?

7. How does stress impact behavior?

8. Explain the relationship of stress to the various diseases.

9. What are the economic and social costs of stress?

10. Characterize several techniques for managing stress.

11. Discuss the behaviors useful in avoiding or reducing stress.

Expert Interviewed

In the video segment of this lesson, the following health professional shares his expertise to help you understand the material presented.

James W. Pennebaker, Ph.D., Professor of Psychology, Southern Methodist University, Dallas, Texas

Video Focus Points

The following questions are designed to help you get the most from the video segment of this lesson. Review them before you watch the video. After viewing the video segment, write responses notes to reinforce what you have learned.

1. Explain and give examples of cataclysmic, personal, and background stressors.

2. What are situational stressors normally defined by the dimensions of health and how can they affect the individual?

3. Describe the body's physiologic response to stress.

4. Discuss several healthy ways to manage and cope with stress.

Individual Health Plan

This portion of the lesson is designed to enable you to apply the information you have learned to your own life situation and improve the quality of your life. You should do any exercise assigned, complete the journal portion of the plan, then put this portion of the health plan into practice in your life.

Using the self-assessment, "How Stressed Are You," in your textbook on pp. 34 and 35, measure your own stress level. In your journal write a brief evaluation of your stress levels and stressors. Using what you have learned in this lesson, develop a plan for managing and reducing the effects of stress in your life.

Enrichment Opportunity

This suggestion guides you if you want more information on this lesson, want to explore new ideas, or if your instructor requires it. If you are doing this section as a course requirement, consult with your instructor for specific guidelines or directions.

List and practice one of the relaxation or other techniques for managing stress.

Practice Test

After reading the assignment and watching the video, you should be able to answer the Practice Test questions. Tests also include essay questions that are similar to the Text Focus Points, the Video Focus Points, and the Objectives. When you have completed the Practice Test questions, turn to the Answer Key to score your answers.

1. Reactions of different individuals to a particular stressor are
   A. unrelated to an individual's background or upbringing.
   B. not affected by other stressors present in a person's life.
   C. under study by stress experts.
   D. often linked to learned thoughts and feelings.

2. The effects of prolonged exposure to chronic stressors are
   A. much less harmful than stress caused by acute stressors.
   B. contributors to difficulty in adapting and to health problems.
   C. rarely alleviated by a network of social support.
   D. not a concern of mental health professionals.

3. The two physiological systems activated by stressors are the
   A. autonomic nervous system and the endocrine system.
   B. digestive system and the respiratory system.
   C. parasympathetic nervous system and the circulatory system.
   D. autonomic nervous system and the adrenal system.

4. Dangerous behavioral reactions to stress include
   A. dependence on drugs and alcohol.
   B. hypertension and heart disease.
   C. progressive relaxation and biofeedback.
   D. increased alertness and quick pulse.

5. Which of the following is a true statement about the link between stress and disease?
   A. Stress has been observed to be highly correlated with certain diseases.
   B. Stress has been proved to be the cause of both heart disease and diabetes.
   C. Stress boosts the ability of the immune system to fight viral infections.
   D. Stress has been shown to be weakly correlated with hypertension.

6. Which of the following best describes job burnout?
   A. Exhaustion caused by overwork and frustration with a job
   B. Resistance to infections because of an immunologic breakdown
   C. Sudden and unexpected increase in creativity and job performance
   D. Routine stress experienced by most workers

7. Healthy behaviors for reducing stress focus on all the following areas EXCEPT
   A. exercise.
   B. nutrition.
   C. muscle-relaxant drugs.
   D. mental outlook.

8. Traffic delays and a busy job are examples of
   A. cataclysmic stress.
   B. personal stress.
   C. background stress.
   D. spiritual stress.

9. Sustained levels of stress, over the long term, have
   A. possible effects on immune function.
   B. proven effect on lifestyles.
   C. only effect on emotional health.
   D. little effect on physiological function.

10. An individual can cope with stresses by allocating some time for relaxation while
    A. eliminating all problems at once.
    B. solving one problem at a time.
    C. ignoring all problems.
    D. trying to stay busier.

11. Stress that has a negative effect on a person is referred to as _____.

12. A person who is impatient and competitive is exhibiting behavior known as _____.

13. The method for relieving muscle tension that moves through the muscle groups of the body is called _____ relaxation.

14. Stressors frequently related to communication problems are _____ stressors.

15. The body adjusts itself to respond to stressors in the _____ stage.

True or False
16. The general adaptation syndrome gains importance from depiction of stress leading to physiological damage.

17. Personality has no affect on the impact of stress on the body.

18. Time management has little value in controlling stress related problems.

19. Personal stressors are intense, powerful situations that affect the individual rather than large groups.

20. The body's physiological response to stress is quite unpredictable and varies from individual to individual.

Answer Key

These are the correct answers with reference to the Learning Objectives, and to the source of the information: the Textbook Focus Points, Levy, *et al. Life and Health,* and the Video Focus Points. Page numbers are also given for the Textbook Focus Points. "KT" indicates questions with Key Terms defined.

Question	Answer	Learning Objective	Textbook Focus Point (page no.)	Video Focus Point
1.	D	2.1	1 (p. 30)	
2.	B	2.1	2 (p. 32)	
3.	A	2.2	5 (p. 36)	
4.	A	2.3	7 (p. 40)	
5.	A	2.3	8 (p. 41)	
6.	A	2.3	9 (p. 44)	
7.	C	2.4	11 (pp. 49-50)	
8.	C	2.1		1
9.	A	2.2		3
10.	B	2.4		4
11.	distress	2.1	3 (p. 33)	KT
12.	Type A	2.2	6 (pp. 37, 39)	KT
13.	progressive	2.4	10 (p. 45)	
14.	social	2.1		2
15.	alarm	2.2		3
16.	T	2.2	4 (p. 33)	
17.	F	2.2	6 (p. 37)	
18.	F	2.4	11 (p. 49)	
19	T	2.1		1
20.	F	2.2		3

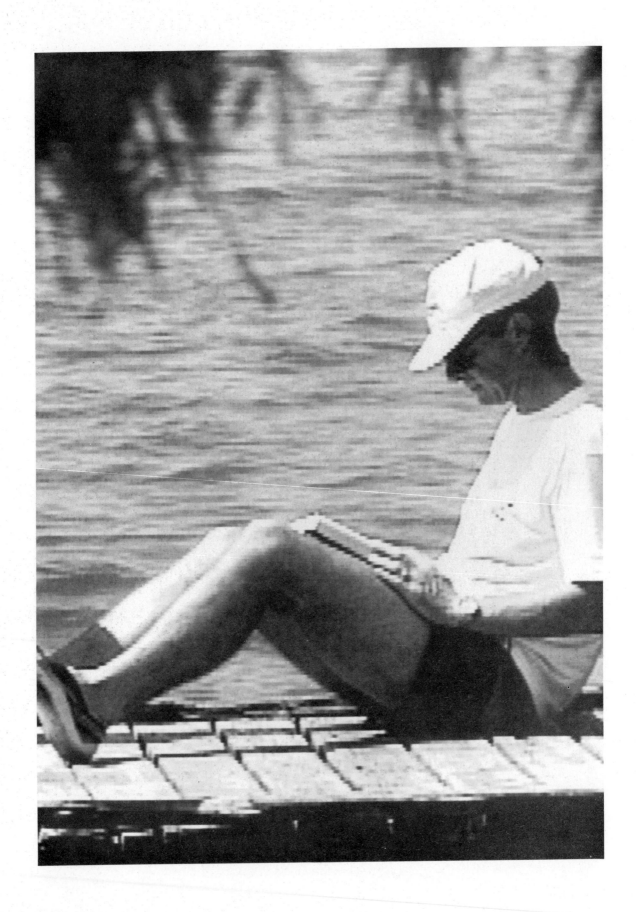

Lesson 3

Emotional Health

Simplification of outward life is not enough. It is merely the outside. But I am starting with the outside. I am looking at the outside of a shell, the outside of my life — the shell. The complete answer is not to be found on the outside, in an outward mode of living. This is only a technique, a road to grace. The final answer, I know, is always inside. But the outside can give a clue, can help one find the inside answer. One is free, like the hermit crab, to change one's shell.

Anne Morrow Lindbergh, *Gift from the Sea*

Overview

When we think of a "healthy" person, we often think first of the physical dimension of health. In reality, our mental health is probably a much more important indicator of our overall health. Our mind lets us feel the range of emotions; love, joy, pleasure, anger, and sadness. If we feel emotionally healthy, we feel better physically, and can cope with physical illness. Our mind defines who we are, sets our goals, determines what we will become, and how happy and satisfying our lives will be.

Our emotions even have a strong physical effect on our bodies. Heart rate, blood volume, blood pressure, electrodermal responses, muscle potential, and brain wave patterns all respond to our emotional state. It is interesting that even though we all experience these physical changes, and label them as emotions, we differ in how we define a particular emotion. One person may feel afraid, while another, experiencing the same physical changes, may feel anger. Again, these examples of our individual differences reflect the ways we learned — by association and by observation.

We all wish our lives would be filled with nothing but positive, happy emotions. In reality, we must frequently deal with negative emotions, conflict, and stress. Anger and anxiety are normal emotions, and most of us have to deal with minor depression occasionally. When we experience these "down" times it is important to remember that there are effective ways to deal with them and turn the negative into a positive. We often use defense mechanisms. These mental strategies protect us from the anxiety associated with painful emotions. We use defense mechanisms to avoid dealing with the painful emotion or problem itself. We may rationalize or deny reality to avoid facing the issue. Some of this is perfectly normal. The trouble comes when we use these too frequently instead of coping with our problems.

Many of us and many of our loved ones will experience emotional disorders at some time. It is important to know that mental health and mental illness are on a continuum with many shadings between extremes. Most emotional problems, like most physical problems, respond well to treatment. Unfortunately, people sometimes are hesitant to seek treatment, or don't recognize the need for treatment, because their thought processes are impaired by the emotional problem. Because, the longer emotional problems go untreated, the more difficult they are to treat, it is important to seek help as soon as the problems are detected.

How do we know if we are emotionally healthy? People who are emotionally healthy have problems, have down times, and sometimes have difficulty coping with their emotions. Yet they can understand and deal with reality. They can adapt to change and cope with stress. They have the capacity for love and concern, and can work effectively to meet their basic needs. If we have these qualities, chances are that we are emotionally healthy.

Learning Objectives

Goal: You should be able to explain the physiology and psychology of emotions, characteristics of emotionally healthy people, defense mechanisms, common emotional disorders, and suicide.

Objectives: Upon completion of this lesson, you should be able to:

1. Explain the basic dimensions of the human mind and the characteristics that emotionally healthy people exhibit.

2. Discuss the physiology and psychology of emotions, explain the negative emotions and how people cope with them, including the use of defense mechanisms.

3. Describe the common emotional disorders, both nonpsychotic and psychotic, and suicide.

Study Assignments

Pay careful attention to the following assignments. The chapter number may not be the same as the lesson number.

Textbook: Chapter 3, "Emotional Health and Intellectual Well-Being," pp. 54-71, 80-81

Video: "Emotional Health"

Key Terms

Watch for these terms and pay particular attention to what each one means, as you follow the textbook and video.

Psychosomatic disease   Panic disorder
Central nervous system   Personality disorder
Peripheral nervous system   Somatoform disorder
Defense mechanism   Psychotic disorder
Nonpsychotic disorder   Major depression
Adjustment disorder   Bipolar disorder
Anxiety disorder   Schizophrenia
Phobia

Textbook Focus Points

Before you read the textbook assignment, review the following points to help focus your thoughts. After you complete the assignment, write out your responses to reinforce what you have learned.

1. Explain the two basic dimensions of the human mind.

2. Identify the two levels of the nervous system and their parts. Explain the physiology and psychology of emotions.

3. What is anxiety? How can a person cope with negative emotions?

4. Describe depressed persons and ways to cope with mild depression. What is the purpose of defense mechanisms? Explain the various defense mechanisms.

5. What is emotional health? What are the basic characteristics that emotionally healthy people exhibit?

6. Describe nonpsychotic disorders. List and explain the common nonpsychotic disorders.

7. List and explain the most frequently occurring psychotic disorders.

8. How can individuals recognize that the risk of suicide exists in themselves or someone else?

Experts Interviewed

In the video segment of this lesson, the following medical professionals share their expertise to help you understand the material presented.

Alvin F. Poussaint, M.D., Senior Associate of Psychiatry, Judge Baker Children's Center, Boston, Massachusetts

Pedro M. Perez, M.D., Medical Director, Children and Adolescent Services, Green Oaks Hospital, Dallas, Texas

Video Focus Points

The following questions are designed to help you get the most from the video segment of this lesson. Review them before you watch the video. After viewing the video segment, write responses to reinforce what you have learned.

1. What are some of the attributes of emotionally healthy people?

2. Describe some of the most common negative emotions and the way in which they can affect the individual.

3. Discuss some of the ways in which emotionally healthy people cope with negative emotions and conflict.

4. Explain the factors that put an individual at risk for suicide. Include the signs that would alert others to the fact that an individual may be thinking of suicide.

Individual Health Plan

This portion of the lesson is designed to enable you to apply the information you have learned to your own life situation and improve the quality of your life. You should do any exercise assigned, complete the journal portion of the plan, then put this portion of the health plan into practice in your life.

> In your journal, keep track of your emotional ups and downs for a week. Write down the situations that affected your emotional state, what actions you took or responses you used, and what the results were. Also list the defense mechanisms you use to avoid emotional pain. Are you surprised at any of your findings? If there are things you would like to change, develop a plan for changing your responses or actions. If you are experiencing much emotional pain or depression, consider seeking professional help.

Enrichment Opportunity

This suggestion guides you if you want more information on this lesson, want to explore new ideas, or if your instructor requires it. If you are doing this section as a course requirement, consult with your instructor for specific guidelines or directions.

> Interview some people that you consider emotionally healthy. Find out something about their lifestyle, and how they cope with problems in life.

Practice Test

After reading the assignment and watching the video, you should be able to answer the Practice Test questions. Tests also include essay questions that are similar to the Text Focus Points, the Video Focus Points, and the Objectives. When you have completed the Practice Test questions, turn to the Answer Key to score your answers.

1. What are the two basic dimensions of the human mind?
   A. Affective and cognitive
   B. Psychological and physiological
   C. Ordered and disordered
   D. Self-concept and self-esteem

2. Which of the following is NOT a physiological response linked to the emotions?
   A. Changes in heart rate
   B. Changes in electrodermal responses
   C. Changes in blood volume
   D. Changes in anxiety

3. Which of the following statements is NOT helpful advice for an individual trying to get over a minor depression?
   A. Make a daily schedule
   B. Acknowledge the source of anger
   C. Direct your energy toward yourself
   D. Exercise regularly

4. Defense mechanisms tend to do all EXCEPT
   A. serve as a means of coping with painful emotions.
   B. act as a temporary buffer to stress.
   C. reduce tension and anxiety.
   D. solve the problem causing the stress.

5. Which of the following characteristics is NOT an indication of good emotional health?
   A. Concern for other people
   B. Ability to work productively
   C. Willingness to adapt to change
   D. Avoidance of extreme emotions

6. An individual who feels recurring episodes of sudden and intense fear is most likely experiencing a
   A. schizoid personality disorder.
   B. panic disorder.
   C. narcissistic personality disorder.
   D. somatoform disorder.

7. An individual who hears voices, is extremely paranoid, and is disconnected from reality is most likely exhibiting a
   A. bipolar disorder.
   B. schizophrenic disorder.
   C. somatic disorder.
   D. nonpsychotic disorder.

8. Warning signs of suicide include all EXCEPT
   A. extreme mood swings.
   B. severe depression.
   C. positive outlook.
   D. talk of death or suicide.

9. Emotionally healthy people
   A. frequently cope with depression.
   B. usually see ways to overcome problems.
   C. never experience failure.
   D. always seem to be happy.

10. That negative emotions affect individuals is evidenced by all the following symptoms EXCEPT
    A. interruptions in sleep.
    B. change in appetite.
    C. feelings of intense despair.
    D. ability to concentrate.

11. Healthy ways of coping with negative emotions would be LEAST likely to include
    A. maintaining self-esteem.
    B. talking to others.
    C. denying the emotions.
    D. doing enjoyable activities.

12. The part of the nervous system which includes the brain and spinal cord, and regulates all body functions is termed _____.

13. A defense mechanism that restricts an individual's conscious awareness of threatening emotions is _____.

14. A person who has lost contact with reality is experiencing a _____.

15. Emotions that disrupt the balance of one's life are termed _____.

16. Feelings of hopelessness, helplessness, and despair can increase the risk of _____.

True or False
17. Negative emotions are a sign of mental disorder.

18. Nonpsychotic disorders distort thoughts and emotions so much that the individual loses contact with reality.

19. Short of seeking professional help, an individual can do little to cope with negative emotions.

20. Being able to talk about feelings of suicide with caring friends can temporarily lower an individual's probability of acting.

Answer Key

These are the correct answers with reference to the Learning Objectives, and to the source of the information: the Textbook Focus Points, Levy, *et al. Life and Health,* and the Video Focus Points. Page numbers are also given for the Textbook Focus Points. "KT" indicates questions with Key Terms defined.

Question	Answer	Learning Objective	Textbook Focus Point (page no.)		Video Focus Point
1.	A	3.1	1 (p. 55)		
2.	D	3.2	2 (pp. 56-58)		
3.	C	3.2	4 (p. 63)		
4.	D	3.2	4 (p. 64)		
5.	D	3.1	5 (p. 65)		
6.	B	3.3	6 (pp. 67-68)	KT	
7.	B	3.3	7 (p. 70)	KT	
8.	C	3.3	8 (pp. 80-81)		
9.	B	3.1			1
10.	D	3.2			2
11.	C	3.2			3
12.	central	3.2	2 (p. 56)	KT	
13.	repression	3.2	4 (p. 64)		
14.	psychotic disorder	3.3	7 (p. 69)	KT	
15.	negative	3.2			2
16.	suicide	3.3			4
17.	F	3.2	3 (p. 60)		
18.	F	3.3	6 (p. 66)	KT	
19.	F	3.2			2
20.	T	3.3			4

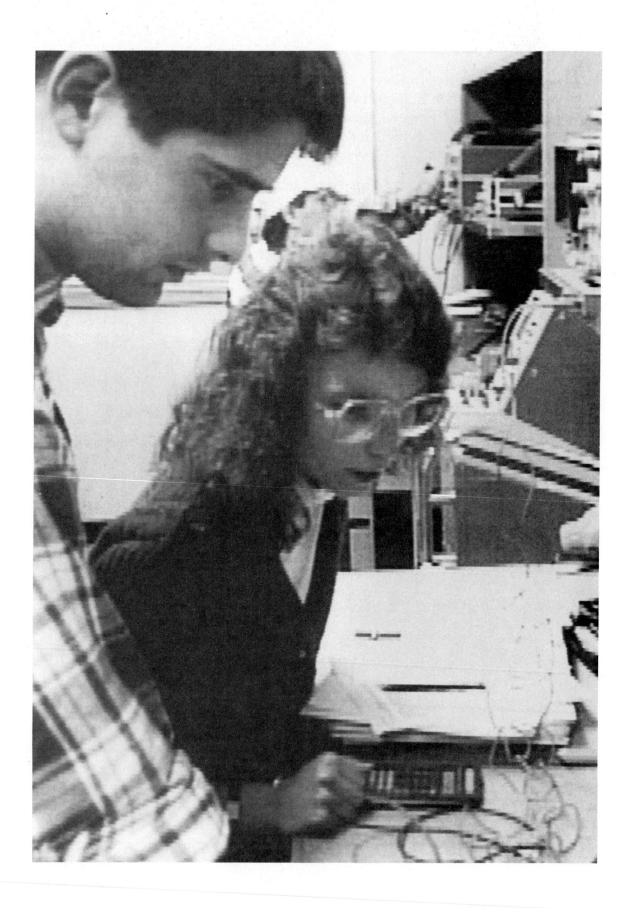

Lesson 4

Intellectual Well-Being

Morale is self-esteem in action.

Avery Weisman, M.D.

Overview

Though many people equate intellect with education, the two are far from the same. Our **intellect** is the thinking, reasoning, problem-solving part of our consciousness. We all have it, no matter what our level of education. While our emotions allow us to feel, our intellect moderates these emotions, and helps us to solve problems and to learn. Our **emotions** and our **intellect** work together to make us mentally healthy. If one or the other is not fully used, we lack quality of life, and can even become mentally ill.

The ability to learn is critical to our health. We begin learning from birth, and continue to learn throughout life. We model the behavior of others. We learn through trial and error, and we remember past experiences. Our behavior and health practices result from what we have learned from our life experiences.

In order to maintain good health, it is imperative that we use our intellect to solve problems and make good decisions about our health. To make these decisions, we must be sure we clearly understand the problem. Too often, we try to solve the problem before we really understand it. Look at life's problems from several directions before you try to solve them. Once we understand the problem, we develop strategies for solving it. An important point here is the knowledge that there is rarely only one solution. We must open our minds to the idea that there are various strategies available to us. We may try one that doesn't work. Don't give up — try another one.

The final stage of problem solving is decision making, a critical part of the process! All of us have known people who couldn't seem to make a decision. They could understand the problem, develop strategies, but just didn't take that final step. People like this are frequently unhappy because

---

31 Intellectual Well-Being

others step in and make their decisions for them. Don't be one of these people. Make your own decisions regarding your health. Then — be sure and take action on your decision!

A most important part of our being is our **self-concept**, or the perception we have about ourselves. Our self-concept evolves throughout our lives, based on our evaluation of ourselves and what other people think. Both our emotions and our intellect play an intertwining role in development of a positive self-concept. Self-concept is crucial to our mental health. If we do not have a realistic, positive self-concept, we are not healthy, no matter how healthy we are physically. In order to have high **self-esteem**, or a good sense of worth and dignity, we must have a positive self-concept. This positive self-concept, with its resulting high self-esteem shapes our **self-efficacy**, the confidence that we have in ourselves to accomplish things in our life and take care of our health.

We have spent time discussing the positive aspects of intellect and emotions, but sometimes, during our lives and those of ones we care about, things don't come together in a positive fashion. For whatever reason, there are problems we can't solve or feelings that we can't cope with. In the past, and sometimes even now, people are hesitant to seek help for mental problems. Somehow, seeking mental help may have a stigma that seeking physical help does not have. This is very unfortunate, because it is crucial for people to seek professional help when they have mental or emotional problems. Good counseling or therapy can aid an individual in returning to a fully functioning, high quality of life. If you or someone you know is experiencing depression, problems with relationships, eating or sleeping problems, mood swings, or other signs of emotional problems, make a decision at once to get help. With help, we can overcome these problems and lead a healthy happy life.

Together, our intellect and emotions are the most powerful tools we have for building and maintaining our healthy lifestyle. It is imperative that we use them well.

Learning Objectives

Goal: You should be able to explain intellect and learning, the problem-solving process, and the role of self-concept and self-esteem.

Objectives: Upon completion of this lesson, you should be able to:

1. Explain learning, memory and cognition; including discussion of the various learning theories, and the problem solving process.

2. Discuss the role of self-concept, self-esteem, and self-efficacy in personality.

3. Describe the signs that warn of mental problems and discuss the types of therapy available to persons with mental problems.

Study Assignments

Pay careful attention to the following assignments. The chapter number may not be the same as the lesson number.

Textbook: Chapter 3, "Emotional Health and Intellectual Well-Being," pp. 71-80

Video: "Intellectual Well-Being"

Key Terms

Watch for these terms and pay particular attention to what each one means, as you follow the textbook and video.

Conditioned response theory	**Self-concept**
Classical conditioning theory	**Self-esteem**
Operant conditioning theory	**Behavior therapy**
Social learning theory	**Organic therapy**

Text Focus Points

Before you read the textbook assignment, review the following points to help focus your thoughts. After you complete the assignment, write out your responses to reinforce what you have learned.

1. Explain the conditioned response theories and discuss their importance in learning.

2. Describe social learning theory. What is memory?

3. What is the intellect? Describe the steps of a problem-solving strategy.

4. How do self-concept and self-esteem relate to our well-being?

5. Describe the various kinds of therapy available to people experiencing mental problems.

Expert Interviewed

In the video segment of this lesson, the following medical professional shares his expertise to help you understand the material presented.

W. Robert Beavers, M.D., Clinical Professor of Psychiatry, University of Texas Southwestern Medical School, Dallas, Texas

Video Focus Points

The following questions are designed to help you get the most from the video segment of this lesson. Review them before you watch the video. After viewing the video segment, write responses to reinforce what you have learned.

1. What role does learning, problem-solving, and decision making play in health and well-being?

2. Discuss self-concept and self-esteem.

3. Why is it important to be able to deal with failure in a positive manner?

Individual Health Plan

This portion of the lesson is designed to enable you to apply the information you have learned to your own life situation and improve the quality of your life. You should do any exercise assigned, complete the journal portion of the plan, then put this portion of the health plan into practice in your life.

> Complete the Self-Assessment, "Assessing Your Self-Esteem," on pp. 74-75, of your textbook. Use the results to help you make some decisions about your health. (HINT: Start focusing on your strengths instead of your weaknesses!)

> Using the journal that you are keeping, note the actions and results that you took in situations affecting your emotional state. Apply the problem solving approach to the situations. Did you really understand the problem or situation clearly? Were there other strategies or responses that you could have used? Analyze your decision or lack of decision in the situation. Would you do the same thing again? How could you improve the outcome? Now apply what you have learned to some problems you are encountering now and keep your knowledge for future use.

Enrichment Opportunity

This suggestion guides you if you want more information on this lesson, want to explore new ideas, or if your instructor requires it. If you are doing this section as a course requirement, consult with your instructor for specific guidelines or directions.

> Visit a community mental health resource, such as a crisis intervention center. Become familiar with the role such resources play in a community.

Practice Test

After reading the assignment and watching the video, you should be able to answer the Practice Test questions. Tests also include essay questions that are similar to the Text Focus Points, the Video Focus Points, and the Objectives. When you have completed the Practice Test questions, turn to the Answer Key to score your answers.

1. According to classical conditioning theory, if two different stimuli are experienced together consistently, an animal will soon react as though
   A. both stimuli should be avoided.
   B. both stimuli were different aspects of the same thing.
   C. only the first stimulus exists.
   D. neither stimulus had ever been experienced.

2. Operant conditioning theorists have discovered that positive reinforcement is
   A. more effective than negative reinforcement.
   B. less effective than negative reinforcement.
   C. effective only when accompanied by negative reinforcement.
   D. effective only in controlling affective disorders.

3. Conditioned response theories have been used to understand
   A. emotional stability.
   B. learning.
   C. psychotic disorders.
   D. electroshock therapy.

4. Albert Bandura's learning model, which states that children learn through imitation, is the basis for
   A. classical conditioning theory.
   B. operant conditioning theory.
   C. social learning theory.
   D. personality theory.

5. The two main components of the intellect are
   A. emotions and defense mechanisms.
   B. reality and fantasy.
   C. learning and application.
   D. memory and cognition.

---

6. What is the first step in careful problem solving?
    A. Selecting suitable strategies
    B. Making decisions
    C. Identifying possible alternatives
    D. Understanding the problem

7. An individual who has a high level of self-efficacy also has
    A. several defense mechanisms.
    B. physical health.
    C. high self-esteem.
    D. affective disorders.

8. Common treatments for emotional problems do NOT include
    A. behavior therapy.
    B. psychotherapy.
    C. electroshock therapy.
    D. organic therapy.

9. Which of the following is NOT an example of organic therapy?
    A. Psychotherapy
    B. Electroconvulsive therapy
    C. Psychosurgery
    D. Drug therapy

10. The final, important step in the problem-solving process is to
    A. select strategies.
    B. make a decision.
    C. act on the decision.
    D. define the problem.

11. Self-concept includes individuals' perceptions of their
    A. lovableness.
    B. partners' abilities.
    C. self-esteem.
    D. strengths and weaknesses.

12. Failure must be viewed as a
    A. step in the learning process.
    B. very personal thing.
    C. reflection of oneself.
    D. sign of not trying hard enough.

13. The conditioning that suggests that different sets of objects or events become grouped in one's mind is _____.

14. The thinking, problem-solving, rational side of human consciousness is the _____.

15. Therapy that attempts to alter a person's symptomatic actions without discovering root causes is known as _____.

16. The intellect is the force that causes people to be able to solve problems and make decisions in the process of _____.

17. Being able to accept credit for a job well done is an example of high _____.

True or False
18. Self-esteem describes a person's feelings of worth and dignity.

19. Using one's intuition is the final, important step in problem solving.

20. People who are expanding their experiences will probably experience some failures.

Answer Key

These are the correct answers with reference to the Learning Objectives, and to the source of the information: the Textbook Focus Points, Levy, *et al. Life and Health,* and the Video Focus Points. Page numbers are also given for the Textbook Focus Points. "KT" indicates questions with Key Terms defined.

Question	Answer	Learning Objective	Textbook Focus Point (page no.)		Video Focus Point
1.	B	4.1	1 (pp. 71-72)		
2.	A	4.1	1 (pp. 71-72)		
3.	B	4.1	1 (p. 71)		
4.	C	4.1	2 (p. 72)	KT	
5.	D	4.1	3 (p. 71)		
6.	D	4.1	3 (p. 73)		
7.	C	4.2	4 (p. 76)		
8.	C	4.3	5 (p. 76)		
9.	A	4.3	5 (pp. 77, 79)		
10.	C	4.1			1
11.	D	4.2			2
12.	A	4.3			3
13.	classical	4.1	1 (p. 71)	KT	
14.	intellect	4.1	3 (p. 71)		
15.	behavior	4.3	5 (p. 7)	KT	
16.	learning	4.1			1
17.	self-esteem	4.2			2
18.	T	4.2	4 (p. 76)	KT	
19.	F	4.1			1
20.	T	4.3			3

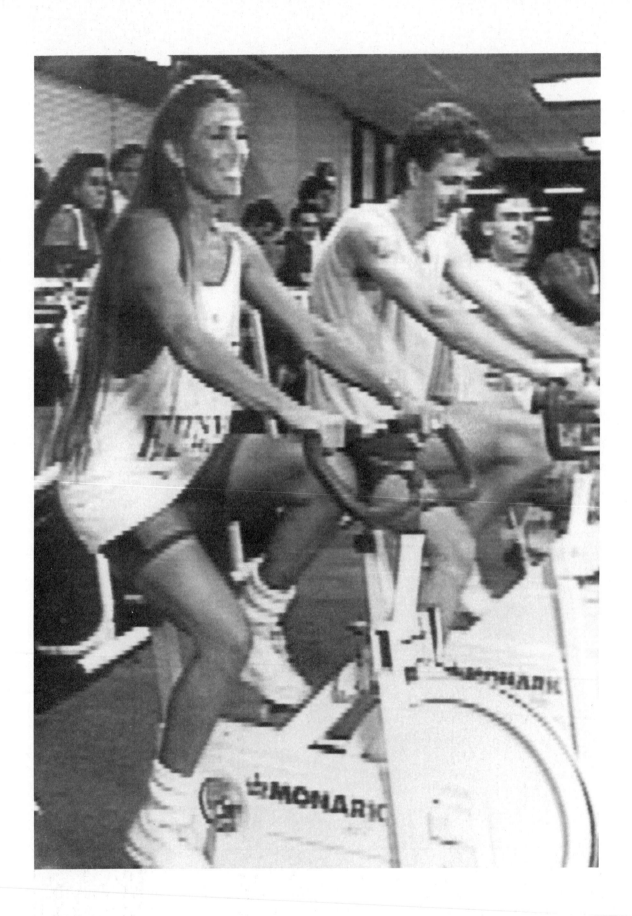

Lesson 5

Fitness and Exercise

You will begin to touch heaven, Jonathon, in the moment that you touch perfect speed. And that isn't flying a thousand miles an hour, or a million, or flying at the speed of light. Because any number is a limit, and perfection doesn't have limits. Perfect speed, my son, is being there.

Richard Bach, *Jonathon Livingston Seagull*

Overview

As the old seagull tells Jonathon, the important thing is being there. So it is with fitness and exercise — the important thing is that you are doing something aerobic on a regular basis. It is not important for you to become a marathon runner, or run the four-minute mile. It is important for you to get enough exercise to keep your cardiovascular system in good shape, and to give you the strength and endurance to do the things you want. It is no secret that people who are physically fit are healthier, more productive, and have a higher quality of life than those who are not. We also know that almost anyone can engage is some kind of exercise program. The mystery is why only about 20 percent of Americans get enough regular exercise.

Some of the answers may lie in our American way of life. We have all kinds of technology to make our life easier. Most of us have sedentary jobs that we drive to and from, and too many of us come home from our sedentary jobs to spend the evening on the couch in front of the television. For recreation, we go to movies or to a spectator sporting event, where the only exercise we get is walking to the concession stand for popcorn. Consider also, this is the model that our children are seeing. Is it any wonder that our "couch potato" image is being passed on to the next generation? We are part of the generation that can change all this, and make ourselves a generation of healthy people, for future generations to model. Besides, **fitness is fun**! It feels good to have the energy to do the things we want to. It is fun to feel in control of this part of our life.

If you are willing to invest even three hours a week in a fitness program, you will see significant results. A program of vigorous walking for 15 to 20 minutes, three times a week, combined with warm-up, stretching, and cool-down activities will accomplish that level of fitness required for good health. If you don't want to or can't walk for exercise, then cycling, swimming, or other aerobic activity will accomplish the same thing. A regular program like this will give you other benefits as well. Exercise helps us cope with stress, makes us feel more healthy emotionally, gives us a feeling of self-esteem and self-efficacy, can be a social activity, and gives our spiritual self a lift as well. This three-hour investment of ourselves helps us achieve all five dimensions of health.

Now that we are all convinced, and ready to start our exercise program, let's discuss the healthy way to start. First, start slowly! If you have been inactive for several years, are more than 30 years old, or suffer from a chronic health problem, examination by a physician is very important. Your physician can order tests that will help ensure that you are ready for an exercise program. If after this lesson you are still unsure how to begin your own program, consult your instructor, a staff member of your college health center, or some other health or physical education professional. The only financial investment that you have to make is in a good pair of suitable shoes designed for the activity you will choose. Remember that just as improvement will begin very soon, conditioning is lost very soon if you stop your program. Make a pledge to yourself to keep your program going. You owe it to yourself!

So, get a checkup, put on those shoes, and hit the road! If you think you might need a little extra motivation and help, enroll in a class at a college near you or join a good fitness club.

Learning Objectives

Goal: You should be able to describe the benefits and principles of exercise, the components of fitness, and explain the components and modifications of an exercise program.

Objectives: Upon completion of this lesson, you should be able to:

1. Describe the physical and psychological benefits of regular exercise, the components of physical fitness, and the principles of exercise.

2. Discuss the components of a plan for a regular exercise program, the modification of the program, and considerations in choosing a place to exercise.

Study Assignments

Pay careful attention to the following assignments. The chapter number may not be the same as the lesson number.

Textbook: Chapter 4, "Activity, Exercise, and Physical Fitness," pp. 85-109

Video: "Fitness and Exercise"

Key Terms

Watch for these terms and pay particular attention to what each one means, as you follow the textbook and video.

Physical activity	**Isokinetic**
Physical exercise	**Isotonic**
Agility	**Isometric**
Balance	**Cardiovascular fitness**
Coordination	**Vital capacity**
Power	**Aerobic exercise**
Reaction time	**Anaerobic exercise**
Speed	**Specificity**
Flexibility	**Overload**
Muscular endurance	**Progression**
Body leanness	**Regularity**
Atrophy	

Text Focus Points

Before you read the textbook assignment, review the following points to help focus your thoughts. After you complete the assignment, write out your responses to reinforce what you have learned.

1. Describe the physical and psychological benefits of regular exercise. Differentiate between activity and exercise. What are some potential risks of exercise, including the experience of sudden pain during exercise?

2. Explain the skill-related and the health-related components of physical fitness. Describe the benefits and techniques of stretching. What should be done before stretching?

3. Distinguish between isokinetic, isotonic, and isometric exercise. What are disadvantages to isotonic exercise programs? Describe the difference between weight-training programs designed to build muscular endurance and those designed to build muscular strength.

4. Define cardiovascular fitness and describe how it improves health. What happens to the heart during exercise?

5. Describe and compare aerobic and anaerobic exercise. Discuss the principles of exercise: specificity, overload, progression, and regularity.

6. Distinguish fitness-for-health plans from fitness-for-skill plans. What are recommendations regarding choosing and beginning a fitness program? What are the recommended goals of a fitness program, and what occurs when a fitness program is not maintained?

7. What are some important points to consider in choosing exercise machines or a health club?

Experts Interviewed

In the video segment of this lesson, the following medical and health professionals share their expertise to help you understand the material presented.

Steven N. Blair, P.E.D., Director of Epidemiology, Cooper Institute for Aerobics Research, Dallas, Texas

Peter G. Snell, Ph.D., Assistant Professor of Medicine and Physiology, University of Texas Southwestern Medical Center, Dallas, Texas

Video Focus Points

The following questions are designed to help you get the most from the video segment of this lesson. Review them before you watch the video. After viewing the video segment, write responses to reinforce what you have learned.

1. What are some of the physical benefits of exercise? Include the components of fitness or, as it is also known, "fitness for health"?

2. What factors need to be considered when designing and beginning an exercise program?

3. In what ways is progression important in an exercise program?

4. Describe some of the mental and emotional benefits of exercising.

Individual Health Plan

This portion of the lesson is designed to enable you to apply the information you have learned to your own life situation and improve the quality of your life. You should do any exercise assigned, complete the journal portion of the plan, then put this portion of the health plan into practice in your life.

> In the journal you are keeping, keep track of your physical activity and your physical exercise for a week or more. From this information, and using what you have learned in this lesson, develop a program of regular exercise for yourself. Write the plan in your journal, so that you are able to modify it as you need to. Once you have developed a plan that suits your needs and abilities, begin or continue your regular exercise program.

Enrichment Opportunities

These suggestions guide you if you want more information on this lesson, want to explore new ideas, or if your instructor requires it. If you are doing this section as a course requirement, consult with your instructor for specific guidelines or directions.

1. Visit several health clubs and fitness facilities and compare and evaluate their programs.

2. Interview several people of varying ages and levels of fitness. Ask them about their fitness programs. What did you think about the components of their program and the quality of it?

Practice Test

After reading the assignment and watching the video, you should be able to answer the Practice Test questions. Tests also include essay questions that are similar to the Text Focus Points, the Video Focus Points, and the Objectives. When you have completed the Practice Test questions, turn to the Answer Key to score your answers.

1. Which of the following is a true statement about physical exercise?
   A. Physical exercise includes only movement that results in expenditure of energy.
   B. Physical exercise requires at least 10 minutes at an activity.
   C. Physical exercise produces muscle stress, which leads to muscle growth.
   D. Physical exercise usually involves repetitive movements.

2. Flexibility refers to the movement of joints
   A. in coordinated effort on opposite sides of the body.
   B. during physical fitness activities.
   C. easily through their full range of motion.
   D. only through the range of motion desired.

3. Weight-training programs which emphasize building muscular endurance should include
   A. only isokinetic exercises.
   B. many repetitions with a low to moderate weight load.
   C. few repetitions with a heavy weight load.
   D. only exercises exceeding 10 minutes.

4. The effects of cardiovascular fitness do NOT include increased
   A. volume of blood.
   B. numbers of red blood cells.
   C. strength and efficiency of the heart.
   D. strain on the heart muscle.

5. The primary difference between aerobic exercise and anaerobic exercise is
   A. oxygen consumption.
   B. demand on muscle tissue.
   C. fatigue factor.
   D. overload.

6. A fitness-for-health plan is primarily designed for
   A. competition athletes.
   B. senior citizens.
   C. basic fitness needs.
   D. young adults to age 20.

7. Which of the following should NOT be used for aerobic conditioning?
   A. Treadmills
   B. Weight stack machines
   C. Rowing machines
   D. Stationary bicycles

8. The components of fitness include all the following EXCEPT
   A. strength.
   B. skill.
   C. endurance.
   D. flexibility.

9. In designing a fitness program, one of the most important considerations is the individual's
   A. initial fitness level.
   B. height.
   C. skill level.
   D. schedule.

10. Progression in an exercise program is important to
    A. maintain health benefits.
    B. improve fitness levels.
    C. increase skill levels.
    D. feel good.

11. Mental benefits of exercise include all the following EXCEPT
    A. sense of well-being.
    B. cardiovascular health.
    C. mental alertness.
    D. positive attitude.

12. Any voluntary body movement that results in an expenditure of energy is physical _____.

13. The ability to exercise the whole body for long periods and have the circulating system supply the fuel to keep the body going is _____.

14. The type of exercise which is sustained at a level that allows the body to meets its oxygen needs is called _____.

15. It is important to design an exercise program that builds endurance, flexibility, and _____.

True or False
16. Balance is the ability to maintain or regain upright posture, or equilibrium, while moving or standing still.

17. If more than one day passes between exercise sessions, "detraining" begins.

18. Belonging to a health club is an important part of a fitness program.

19. Progression in an exercise program is just one of the ways to increase fitness level.

20. While increased physical fitness is a benefit of exercise, emotional benefits must come from other activities.

Answer Key

These are the correct answers with reference to the Learning Objectives, and to the source of the information: the Textbook Focus Points, Levy, *et al. Life and Health,* and the Video Focus Points. Page numbers are also given for the Textbook Focus Points. "KT" indicates questions with Key Terms defined.

Question	Answer	Learning Objective	Textbook Focus Point (page no.)		Video Focus Point
1.	D	5.1	1 (p. 87)	KT	
2.	C	5.1	2 (p. 90)	KT	
3.	B	5.1	3 (p. 95)		
4.	D	5.1	4 (pp. 95-96)		
5.	A	5.1	5 (p. 97)		
6.	C	5.2	6 (p. 101)		
7.	B	5.2	7 (p. 105)		
8.	B	5.1			1
9.	A	5.2			2
10.	B	5.2			3
11.	B	5.1			4
12.	activity	5.1	1 (p. 87)	KT	
13.	cardiovascular fitness	5.1	4 (p. 95)	KT	
14.	aerobic	5.1	5 (p. 96	KT	
15.	strength	5.2			2
16.	T	5.1	2 (p. 90)	KT	
17.	F	5.2	6 (p. 103)		
18.	F	5.2	7 (p. 105)		
19.	F	5.2			3
20.	F	5.1			4

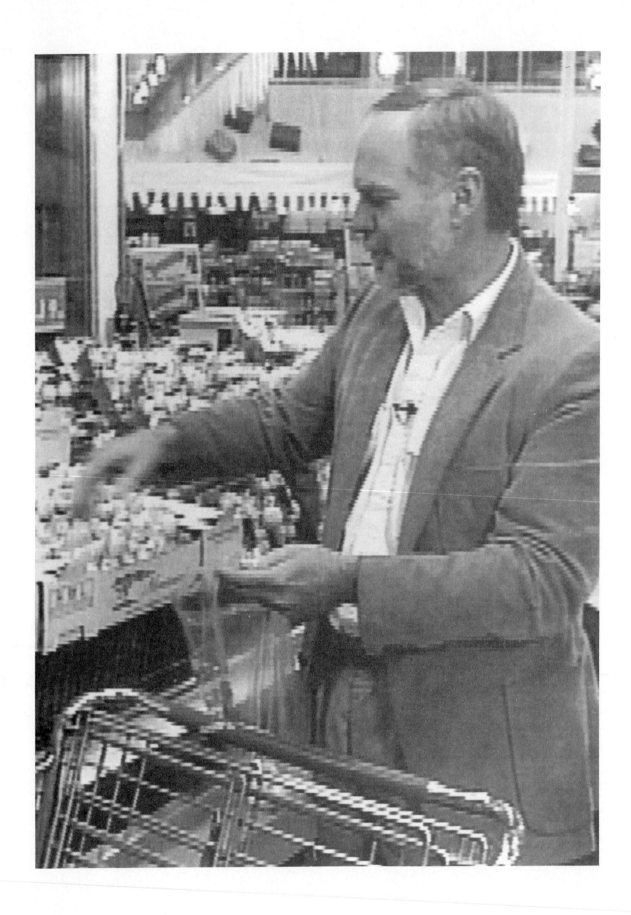

Lesson 6

Diet and Nutrition

We're not sure whether vegetables are macho enough.

Arlyn Hackett

Overview

We probably think more about diet and nutrition today than ever before in our history. However, do we really practice better nutrition principles now that we know what we should be eating? If we look at the crowds in local farmer's markets buying fresh fruit and vegetables, we would say yes. However if we check out the lines in the neighborhood fast food establishments, the answer would be absolutely not. Then, if we followed you around the grocery store, the answer would be ????

Thanks to advanced technology, higher standard of living, and an abundance of nutrition information, we have access to very good nutrition. Yet, for a variety of reasons, many of us are malnourished. We certainly eat plenty; frequently too much. Unfortunately, too often we make poor choices in our selection of food. We tend to eat foods that are high in saturated fat, salt, and refined sugar, rather than choosing fruits, vegetables, and foods high in fiber and low in fats. Even worse, children eat just like adults, thus increasing their risk of nutrition-related illness.

Many people complain that good nutrition is expensive or too much trouble. Actually, a healthy diet can be far less expensive than a poor one and just as easy to prepare. Fast food and "junk" food are certainly not cheap. Few of the rich, refined foods are easy to prepare. Good nutrition involves an understanding of foods that are healthy, and some simple planning of daily intake. Plainly stated, we need to increase our consumption of complex carbohydrates, decrease our consumption of protein, and limit our fats, salt, and refined sugar. Translated into foods, this means more fruits, vegetables, whole grain and enriched breads and pasta, and less meats, eggs, salt, fats, and high calorie desserts. It also means steaming, baking, or broiling foods instead of frying them or covering them with gravy or rich sauces.

Even those who eat out can improve their nutritional status by using good judgement in food selection. Most restaurants (even our favorite-fast food establishments) are beginning to offer more health conscious options on their menu. The more we choose and request these healthy foods, the more will be offered. All of us can eat a more healthy diet and enjoy it. We can get these foods in most supermarkets and restaurants. We do not need to go to extremes of shopping at a health food store to ensure good nutrition.

We have all the elements of a healthy diet that ensures good nutrition easily available to us if we simply make good choices. You know what to eat — the choice is now yours!

Learning Objectives

Goal: You should be able to discuss nutrition, the components of food, and the principles, strategies, and food choices involved in achieving a healthy diet.

Objectives: Upon completion of this lesson, you should be able to:

1. Explain the term "nutrition" and discuss the components of food including macronutrients, micronutrients, fiber, and water.

2. Discuss various approaches used to achieve a balanced diet, basic principles, strategies, and skills important in achieving good nutrition, and food choices important under special circumstances.

Study Assignments

Pay careful attention to the following assignments. The chapter number may not be the same as the lesson number.

Textbook: Chapter 5, "Diet and Nutrition," pp. 111-137

Video: "Diet and Nutrition"

Key Terms

Watch for these terms and pay particular attention to what each one means, as you follow the textbook and video.

Nutrition	**Unsaturated fat**
Macronutrient	**Saturated fat**
Micronutrient	**Minerals**
Protein	**Calcium**
Essential amino acid	**Potassium**
Complete protein	**Sodium**
Incomplete protein	**Electrolytes**
Carbohydrate	**Iron**
Glucose	**Water-soluble vitamins**
Lipids	**Biochemical individuality**
Cholesterol	**Fat-soluble vitamins**

Text Focus Points

Before you read the textbook assignment, review the following points to help focus your thoughts. After you complete the assignment, write out your responses to reinforce what you have learned.

1. What is meant by the term "nutrition"? What do calories measure and what determines an individual's caloric needs?

2. Distinguish between macronutrients, micronutrients, and essential nonnutritives.

3. How are proteins used by the body? Distinguish between complete and incomplete proteins and identify the sources of food for each. What occurs if there is a deficiency or excess amount of protein in the body?

4. How are carbohydrates, in the form of glucose, used in the body? What are the sources of carbohydrates and in what foods can simple and complex carbohydrates be found? What percent of our calories should come from carbohydrates?

Diet and Nutrition

5. How are fats used by the body? In what amounts can fat be stored in the body and how can stored fats be used? Distinguish between saturated and unsaturated fats. What are the risks involved in consuming cholesterol and saturated fats? What is the recommended intake of saturated fat?

6. Identify the primary food sources of calcium and describe the potential consequences of calcium deficiency. List the primary electrolytes and explain their function. What may cause a decrease in the body's supply of potassium? What is a potential consequence of high sodium intake? Explain the importance of iron and describe who is at greatest risk of iron deficiency and why.

7. What is the overall function of vitamins? Describe the benefits of vitamins A and C. Discuss toxicity as it relates to water-soluble and fat-soluble vitamins. Are vitamin supplements necessary for everyone?

8. What is fiber made of? How does fiber aid in digestion? List sources of fiber. What are the functions of water to the body? How much water should we drink each day?

9. Discuss the various approaches used to achieve a balanced diet. Include positive and negative aspects of each.

10. Describe some of the food choices needed in special situations, such as by vegetarians, and people under stress.

11. Explain strategies and skills important in buying and preparing food, and for eating out. Include the basic universal principles for everyone.

Expert Interviewed

In the video segment of this lesson, the following health professional shares his expertise to help you understand the material presented.

Arlyn Hackett, Chef, Director of Chef Arlyn Hackett's Kitchen, A Cooking School in San Diego, California, Host, PBS series *Health Smart Gourmet Cooking*

Video Focus Points

The following questions are designed to help you get the most from the video segment of this lesson. Review them before you watch the video. After viewing the video segment, write responses to reinforce what you have learned.

1. What are important "tips" or principles for menu planning and selecting food wisely in the supermarket?

2. What is meant by the idea of "reordering the American diet"?

3. Discuss ways in which food can be prepared to lower the intake of fats, salt, and refined sugar and to increase it's nutrition.

Individual Health Plan

This portion of the lesson is designed to enable you to apply the information you have learned to your own life situation and improve the quality of your life. You should do any exercise assigned, complete the journal portion of the plan, then put this portion of the health plan into practice in your life.

In your journal, keep track of your dietary intake for a week. Evaluate it. Is this your normal diet? How do you rank yourself on your intake of healthy foods? Does your diet contain too much cholesterol and saturated fats, salt, sugar, and "empty" calories? Using this evaluation, plan a food strategy that will provide you with good nutrition, and that you will be willing to follow for an extended time.

Once you have written your plan, try it out for two weeks. Reevaluate it and consider making this a permanent part of your lifestyle.

Enrichment Opportunities

These suggestions guide you if you want more information on this lesson, want to explore new ideas, or if your instructor requires it. If you are doing this section as a course requirement, consult with your instructor for specific guidelines or directions.

1. Go to a grocery store and observe what people are buying. Compare and evaluate the quality of their diet, based on their food selections.

2. Go to a cafeteria or buffet and observe how people are eating. Note whether the children are eating like their parents. Evaluate their diet as though they eat all the time as you are seeing them eat now.

Practice Test

After reading the assignment and watching the video, you should be able to answer the Practice Test questions. Tests also include essay questions that are similar to the Textbook Focus Points, the Video Focus Points, and the Objectives. When you have completed the Practice Test questions, turn to the Answer Key to score your answers.

1. Calories are used to measure
    A. percentage of fat in foods.
    B. protein potential of foods.
    C. nutritional value of foods.
    D. energy potential of foods.

2. The macronutrients found in food include all the following EXCEPT
    A. fiber.
    B. proteins.
    C. fats.
    D. carbohydrates.

3. Complete proteins are NOT found in
   A. meat.
   B. eggs.
   C. milk products.
   D. vegetables.

4. Which of the following foods is NOT rich in carbohydrates?
   A. Potatoes
   B. Wheat
   C. Fish
   D. Fruit

5. The only macronutrient that the body can store in large amounts is
   A. protein.
   B. carbohydrate.
   C. fat.
   D. water.

6. What do electrolytes do?
   A. They carry information to the nucleic acids.
   B. They reverse the electrical charges of proteins.
   C. They carry the electrical charges needed by cells.
   D. They transmit genetic information between cells.

7. Why is toxicity rare in water-soluble vitamins?
   A. The body can excrete excess amounts.
   B. The body stores excess amounts.
   C. The body converts excess amounts into carbohydrates.
   D. The body converts excess amounts into fatty acids.

8. What are the basic four food groups?
   A. Meat, milk products, fruits and vegetables, and breads and cereals
   B. Amino acids, fatty acids, electrolytes, and triglycerides
   C. Macronutrients, micronutrients, vitamins, and minerals
   D. Vitamins, minerals, fiber, and water

9. Which of the following is a true statement about following a vegetarian diet?
    A. Vegetarian diets contain more necessary nutrients than do ovolacto diets.
    B. Vegetarian diets will not contain all the necessary amino acids.
    C. Vegetarian diets do not include proteins.
    D. Vegetarian diets often combine foods such as rice and beans to create complete proteins.

10. Healthy nutrition and food selection
    A. becomes quite expensive.
    B. involves careful choices.
    C. seems difficult to achieve.
    D. tends to be boring.

11. Americans typically eat meals that contain too few
    A. meat products.
    B. breads.
    C. milk products.
    D. vegetables.

12. In recent years there has been a great deal of concern about the relationship between high blood pressure and the mineral _____.

13. Coming in forms such as corn syrup and molasses, the most widely used food additive is _____.

14. When evaluating meat and dairy products, of particular concern are the calories that come from _____.

15. One of the healthiest ways to prepare vegetables is _____.

True or False
16. Nutrition is the process by which the nutrients in food are converted into body tissue and energy.

17. The body can survive much longer without food than without water.

18. Eating foods that are high in nutrition is expensive.

19. It is important to begin to consider vegetables and grains, instead of meat, as the primary focus of the plate.

20. Herbs and spices contain so much sodium that they are not a good substitute for salt.

Answer Key

These are the correct answers with reference to the Learning Objectives, and to the source of the information: the Textbook Focus Points, Levy, *et al. Life and Health,* and the Video Focus Points. Page numbers are also given for the Textbook Focus Points. "KT" indicates questions with Key Terms defined.

Question	Answer	Learning Objective	Textbook Focus Point (page no.)	Video Focus Point
1.	D	6.1	1 (p. 112)	
2.	A	6.1	2 (p. 112)	KT
3.	D	6.1	3 (p. 113)	
4.	C	6.1	4 (p. 115)	
5.	C	6.1	5 (p. 115)	
6.	C	6.1	6 (p. 119)	KT
7.	A	6.1	7 (p. 121)	
8.	A	6.2	9 (p. 124)	
9.	D	6.2	10 (p. 130)	
10.	B	6.2		1
11.	D	6.2		2
12.	sodium	6.1	6 (p. 119)	
13.	sugar	6.2	11 (p. 133)	
14.	fat	6.2		1
15.	steaming	6.3		3
16.	F	6.1	1 (p. 112)	KT
17.	T	6.1	8 (p. 123)	
18.	F	6.2		1
19.	T	6.2		2
20.	F	6.3		3

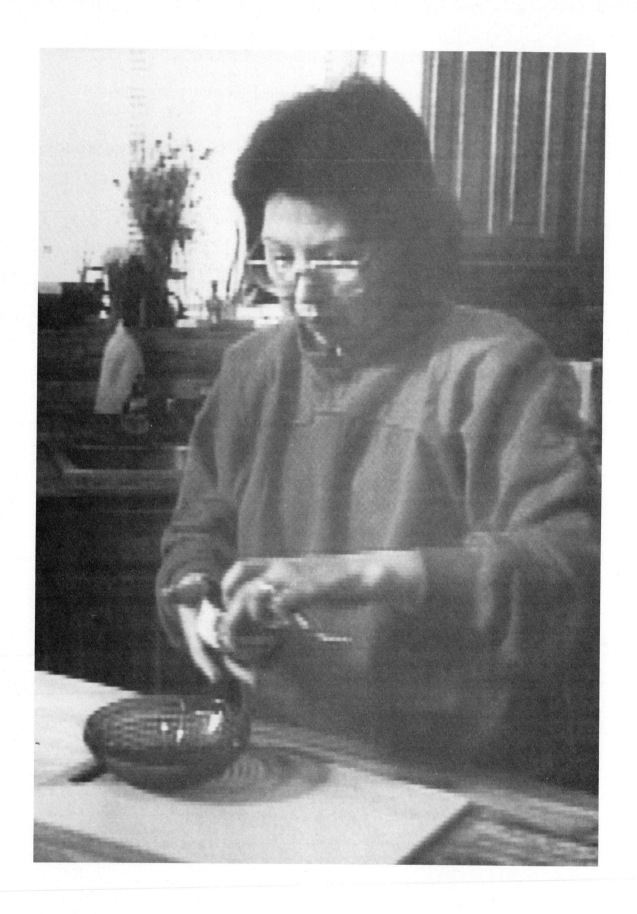

Lesson 7

Weight Management

Some weight-loss plans are based on poor science or no science, and many on witchcraft.

Peter D. Wood, Ph. D.

Overview

Have you noticed how many new diet books are being written, and how every magazine on the newsstand has a diet article every month? Does that tell you something? Americans are obsessed with dieting and everything that goes with it. Many people try every fad diet that comes out, only to lose the same twenty or thirty pounds over and over in a yo-yo pattern that gets them nowhere. Most of the fad diets are useless in the long run, and many are actually dangerous.

The obsession with thinness has even given us two relatively new disease conditions related to diet and self-concept: anorexia nervosa and bulimia. Both are fairly new to medicine and are a result of an obsession with thinness. These are very serious problems which have resulted in many deaths, particularly in young women.

There are many reasons for overweight, and we know that obesity raises our risks for many health problems. Most of us who are overweight know this, and are concerned with how to lose the excess weight and keep it off. The "bottom line" for how to do this is that we must expend more calories than we take in, and do so in a healthy way. We must also change our eating patterns and our lifestyle over the long term, and not simply think in terms of weeks or months. We must also believe that we can do it. This is a matter of self-efficacy and self-esteem.

The key to losing weight and keeping it off is very familiar to all of us — a well balanced diet, low in fats and simple sugars combined with a good exercise program. If that sounds familiar, it should. The same fruits, vegetables, fiber, and complex carbohydrates that are essential to good nutrition are the drivers for a healthy weight loss diet. We should be

---

eating the healthy foods recommended for good nutrition, and be leaving off the high calorie, high fat, and empty calorie foods that increase our weight and cholesterol levels. Along with this, a sound exercise program is essential. Remember what we learned about expending more calories than we take in! There is no doubt that explaining the principles of weight management is simpler than actually doing it. But once you get started, it gets easier. It also helps to take it one day at a time, but know you are making lifestyle changes for the long term.

It is very important not to be misled by fad diets that promise quick weight loss or magic results. These only get you into trouble. What you are trying to accomplish is a relatively steady weight loss of one to two pounds a week, and an increase in your fitness level through your exercise program.

A very important thing to remember in all this is that your value as a person is **not** related to how much you weigh! Yes, you will be happier and healthier if you attain your goals in body composition and fitness level, but do not let this be the thing that you base your whole self-concept on. If you truly believe your value as a person is unrelated to your body composition, you will actually have an easier time with weight loss.

For those who are underweight, the same basic principles apply. In order to gain weight in a healthy way, you should increase your intake of the starchy foods in a diet based on good nutrition. You should still avoid the high protein or high fat diets, which can be dangerous. Exercise is a key to this program as well.

The principles you are learning apply whether you are overweight, underweight, or just right. A nutritious, well-balanced diet combined with a good exercise program is important for everyone.

Learning Objectives

Goal: You should be able to discuss body composition, body composition problems, and the successful control of body composition.

Objectives: Upon completion of this lesson, you will be able to:

1. Explain body composition, and the relationship of body composition to physical, emotional, and social health.

2. Describe the nature and types of fat, the measures of body composition, and the pull and the push schools for understanding body composition problems. Include discussion of weight and eating disorders.

3. Discuss the common approaches to body composition management, and components necessary for successful body composition management.

Study Assignments

Pay careful attention to the following assignments. The chapter number may not be the same as the lesson number.

Textbook: Chapter 6, "Weight Management and Body Composition," pp. 138-166

Video: "Weight Management"

Key Terms

Watch for these terms and pay particular attention to what each one means, as you follow the textbook and video.

Body composition	Push school
Essential fat	Short-term regulatory mechanism
Storage fat	Long-term regulatory mechanism
Hydrostatic weighing	Setpoint theory
Bioelectrical impedance	Basal metabolism
Skinfold measurement	Externality theory
Fat grafting	Anorexia nervosa
Liposuction	Bulimia
Pull school	

Text Focus Points

Before you read the textbook assignment, review the following points to help focus your thoughts. After you complete the assignment, write out your responses to reinforce what you have learned.

1. What is meant by the term body composition? Explain the relationship of body composition to physical, emotional, and social health.

2. Describe the function and storage areas of essential and storage fat. Define and state the limitations of the three popular methods of body composition measurement. What are the principles these methods are based on?

3. Describe health problems associated with the following types of diet: low calorie, extreme restriction of macronutrients, and formula diets. Describe the criteria for a good diet. Describe the effects of anaerobic and aerobic exercise on body composition. What are the consequences of using laxatives or diuretics for weight loss? Describe liposuction and fat grafting procedures and their consequences. Who are most likely to benefit from group weight loss programs and what are key elements of success?

4. Explain the pull school and the push school as approaches to understanding body composition problems.

5. What is the basic principle of weight regulation? Describe the components necessary for successful control of body composition.

6. Discuss the various weight disorders and eating disorders. How should extreme obesity be treated?

Experts Interviewed

In the video segment of this lesson, the following health professionals share their expertise to help you understand the material presented.

Toni Beck, M.A., Tom Landry Sports Medicine and Research Center, Dallas, Texas

Joseph H. McVoy, Jr., Ph. D., Director, Association for the Health Enrichment of Large People, Director, Eating Disorders Program, Saint Albans Psychiatric Hospital, Radford, Virginia

Peter D. Wood, D.Sc., Ph. D., Professor of Medicine and Associate Director, Stanford Center for Research in Disease Prevention, Stanford University, Palo Alto, California

Video Focus Points

The following questions are designed to help you get the most from the video segment of this lesson. Review them before you watch the video. After viewing the video segment, write responses to reinforce what you have learned.

1. Explain the various aspects of the risks of overweight. What are some of the causes of overweight?

2. Describe some considerations in planning a weight loss diet.

3. Why is exercise important in weight management? What kind of exercise program should be designed?

4. Discuss the causes and dangers of anorexia nervosa and bulimia.

Individual Health Plan

This portion of the lesson is designed to enable you to apply the information you have learned to your own life situation and improve the quality of your life. You should do any exercise assigned, complete the journal portion of the plan, then put this portion of the health plan into practice in your life.

Using the Self-Assessment on page 143 of your text, evaluate your body composition. Using the calculating chart on page 156, of your text, compute the number of calories your body is using to maintain your present weight. Using your diet for the week from your journal, as well as your exercise plan, evaluate your need to change your body composition in some way, or to change your exercise plan. In your journal write some notes on your lifestyle patterns of eating and exercising — when you eat, what makes you want to eat

---

more or less, what interrupts your exercise routine, etc. Also use a mirror to do an evaluation of what you see. (Remember: we are not putting a value on you as a person here — just evaluating body composition.) Are there things you need or want to change for better health? Include these in your journal entry. Now, write out a realistic plan for yourself to manage your body composition. When you have done this, try it out for a few weeks. Evaluate your progress. If you need to, make modifications, or get some advice from a professional. Now keep it up! You will be happy you did.

Enrichment Opportunities

These suggestions guide you if you want more information on this lesson, want to explore new ideas, or if your instructor requires it. If you are doing this section as a course requirement, consult with your instructor for specific guidelines or directions.

1. Compare the nutritional value of several different fad diets to one based on good nutrition. Evaluate your findings.

2. Visit several weight loss centers and find out about their programs. Compare them and evaluate your findings.

3. Talk to someone who is recovering from or fighting anorexia nervosa or bulimia. Ask them about their perceptions of their problem, their self-concept, their goal for weight, etc.

Practice Test

After reading the assignment and watching the video, you should be able to answer the Practice Test questions. Tests also include essay questions that are similar to the Text Focus Points, the Video Focus Points, and the Objectives. When you have completed the Practice Test questions, turn to the Answer Key to score your answers.

1. Overweight individuals are at an increased risk for developing
   A. heart disease.
   B. low blood pressure.
   C. bone tissue.
   D. eustress.

2. Without essential fat, the body would not be able to
   A. breathe.
   B. metabolize nutrients effectively.
   C. transfer genetic information from cell to cell.
   D. feel pain.

3. What is the theory behind hydrostatic weighing?
   A. Fat is lighter and more buoyant than lean tissue.
   B. Fat is heavier and less buoyant than lean tissue.
   C. Fat is mostly located along the skin and away from the skeleton.
   D. Fat is mostly located along the skeleton and away from the skin.

4. Most dietitians advise that a healthy and realistic weight-loss goal is to lose between
   A. 1 and 2 pounds per week.
   B. 3 and 5 pounds per week.
   C. 6 and 8 pounds per week.
   D. 8 and 10 pounds per week.

5. Which of the following best supports the pull school of thought?
   A. Thin people eat consciously.
   B. People can begin to associate food with emotions such as happiness and love.
   C. Adopted children often reflect the weight patterns of their biological parents.
   D. Eating behavior can be modified through group programs.

6. If energy intake is less than energy expenditure, the result will be the
   A. loss of weight.
   B. gain of weight.
   C. yo-yo effect.
   D. establishment of a setpoint.

7. Which of the following statements is true of anorexia nervosa?
   A. Most people with anorexia come from upper- or middle-class homes.
   B. Men suffer from anorexia as frequently as do women but hide the condition more effectively.
   C. Most people with anorexia have never been overweight.
   D. Anorexia primarily affects older women.

8. Reasons for overweight include all the following EXCEPT
   A. availability of fatty food.
   B. increased health knowledge.
   C. sedentary lifestyle.
   D. modern technology.

9. In planning a diet to lose weight, it is important to consider all the following EXCEPT
   A. reducing the fastest way.
   B. losing weight gradually.
   C. increasing exercise.
   D. maintaining weight loss.

10. Exercise is important to a weight loss program because of all the following EXCEPT
    A. metabolism is increased.
    B. energy level is improved.
    C. lethargy is increased.
    D. body shape is improved.

11. An important causal factor associated with anorexia nervosa and bulimia is
    A. overweight.
    B. low self-esteem.
    C. lack of appetite.
    D. underweight.

12. Fat that is necessary for the body's normal physiological functioning is _____.

13. The regulatory mechanism which signals the body when to eat is referred to as _____.

14. An individual who experiences eating binges followed by purges suffers from _____.

15. Two major causes of obesity are diets high in fat and lifestyles that are _____.

16. A weight management program must include not only dietary modifications but also _____.

True or False

17. Body composition is the most important measure of a person's character.

18. Anaerobic exercise is as effective as aerobic exercise for achieving weight loss.

19. The very underweight person should eat high-protein or high-fat diets to gain weight.

20. A successful weight loss program involves long term dietary changes.

Answer Key

These are the correct answers with reference to the Learning Objectives, and to the source of the information: the Textbook Focus Points, Levy, *et al. Life and Health,* and the Video Focus Points. Page numbers are also given for the Textbook Focus Points. KT indicates questions with Key Terms defined.

Question	Answer	Learning Objective	Textbook Focus Point (page no.)	Video Focus Point
1.	A	7.1	1 (p. 140)	
2.	B	7.2	2 (p. 142)	
3.	A	7.2	2 (p. 144)	
4.	A	7.3	3 (p. 146)	
5.	C	7.2	4 (p. 151)	
6.	A	7.3	5 (p. 155)	
7.	A	7.2	6 (p. 160)	
8.	B	7.1		1
9.	A	7.3		2
10.	C	7.3		3
11.	B	7.2		4
12.	essential	7.2	2 (p. 142)	KT
13.	short-term	7.2	4 (p. 151)	KT
14.	bulimia	7.2	6 (p. 162)	KT
15.	sedentary	7.1		1
16.	exercise	7.3		3
17.	F	7.1	1 (p. 141)	
18.	F	7.3	3 (p. 148)	
19.	F	7.3	5 (p. 159)	
20.	T	7.3		2

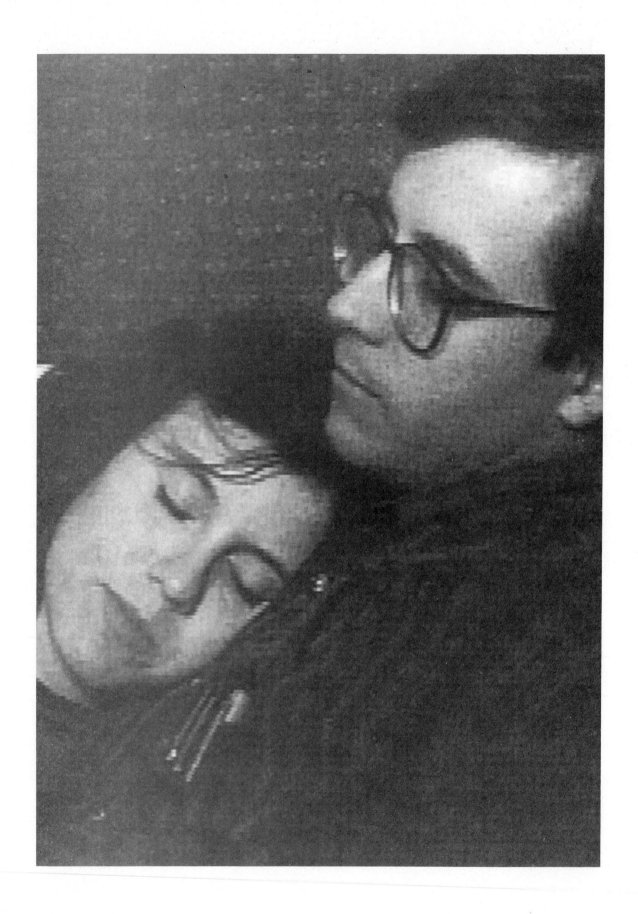

Lesson 8

Intimate Relationships

The pure relationship, how beautiful it is! How easily it is damaged, or weighed down with irrelevancies — not even irrelevancies, just life itself, the accumulations of life and of time. For the first part of every relationship is pure, whether it be friend or lover, husband or child. It is pure, simple, and unencumbered. It is like the artist's vision before he has to discipline it into form, or like the flower of love before it has ripened into the firm but heavy fruit of responsibility. ... Two people listening to each other, two shells meeting each other, making one world between them. There are no others in the perfect unity of that instant, no other people or things or interests. It is free of ties or claims, unburdened by responsibilities, by worry about the future or debts to the past.

Anne Morrow Lindbergh, *Gift from the Sea*

Overview

Think about the relationships you have had in your life. How many truly intimate relationships have you had? How many people do you know with whom you can share your deepest secrets, your true feelings, and innermost thoughts? How many people share this intimate climate of trust and acceptance with you? Not very many? This is not surprising, though you may be surprised when you actually think about it. We all need this nurturance, acceptance, and trust; in a word, intimacy. Yet it may be difficult to attain, and complex to maintain. We first experience intimacy with our parents, then grow to other close relationships with siblings and friends, then develop romantic relationships. For many of us, marriage is the most intimate relationship of all. Throughout our lives we need intimacy, though our intimate relationships with others change as we grow and change. In order to attain intimacy with another, we must have positive self-esteem, self-efficacy, feelings of caring, sharing, trust, commitment and tenderness toward that person. In other words, we must truly care deeply about that person, whether the person is a best friend or lover. In a good marriage the partners may be best friends **and** lovers, but all intimate relationships are by no means sexual ones. Some of the most powerful intimacy is seen in life-long friends.

Developing an intimate romantic relationship, choosing a mate, making the decision to commit to that person, and sustaining a long-term intimate relationship requires much work, but is worth whatever effort we put into it. Too often, we "fall in love" without much thought or concern about the commitment we must be willing to make to sustain the relationship. That intense romantic love that brings us together can rarely be sustained as the years go by, so we must have the deep trust, sharing, affection, and togetherness that is the companionate love that sustains the long-term relationship or marriage.

Though most people marry, there are other very normal lifestyle such as single living and cohabitation. The same need for intimacy is present in people living in these lifestyles. The cohabiting couple is very similar to the married couple in the characteristics and needs of the intimate relationship. The single person may have more difficulty finding those intimate relationships, but certainly needs intimate friends just as do all of us.

Some of the most dramatic changes in the nature of relationships have come in the form of marriages that end with divorce. In the past the idea of "till death do us part" was taken quite literally. People stayed in unhappy marriages for a variety of reasons, frequently because they felt it was better for the children. People today are much less willing to stay in a relationship if they are not getting along and the relationship is not a happy one. While divorce is difficult for everyone involved, it can be a positive solution to a serious relationship problem.

Far worse than any divorce is the occurrence of violence in a relationship. Domestic violence is an alarming problem that affects all segments of the population. The outbreak of violence or abuse in a relationship signifies major problems that must be dealt with professionally. It is absolutely essential that the victim take action to get out of the situation before the violence moves to tragedy.

Building and sustaining an lasting intimate relationship requires us to first have a sense of our own identity, then to be willing to share, to give and receive love, to communicate effectively, and most of all to truly commit to that person and the relationship.

Learning Objectives

Goal: You should be able to discuss the characteristics of and importance of intimate relationships, problems that may develop in intimate relationships, and the components necessary to developing and sustaining intimate relationships.

Objectives: Upon completion of this lesson, you should be able to:

1. Define intimacy, explain the individual's need for it, factors and individual characteristics necessary to developing and sustaining an intimate relationship, and the problems that can arise in an intimate relationship.

2. Explain the concept of love, attraction, and romance in marriage, why people marry, the importance of assessing compatibility in a potential partner, and some alternatives to marriage.

3. Discuss the trends and effects of divorce and domestic violence as outcomes of failed intimate relationships.

Study Assignments

Pay careful attention to the following assignments. The chapter number may not be the same as the lesson number.

Textbook: Chapter 7, "Marriage, Family, and Other Intimate Relationships," pp. 169-178, 185-187, 188-195

Video: "Intimate Relationships"

Key Terms

Watch for these terms and pay particular attention to what each one means, as you follow the textbook and video.

Romantic love
Companionate love
Cohabitation

Textbook Focus Points

Before you read the textbook assignment, review the following points to help focus your thoughts. After you complete the assignment, write out your responses to reinforce what you have learned.

1. Define intimacy, explain the individual's need for intimate relationships, and the factors necessary to developing an intimate relationship.

2. Why do people marry? What are the essential qualities of love? Distinguish between romantic and companionate love. How does a person assess compatibility in a potential partner? How do men's and women's attitudes toward sex differ?

3. Describe the attitudes, trends, and alternatives to marriage.

4. How has the divorce rate changed in recent years? Discuss the effect of divorce on the family members.

5. Discuss the issue of family violence. What are some of the important factors related to the incidence of family violence?

6. Describe some of the qualities that a person must bring to a relationship in order to build a successful intimate relationship. Include some of the issues that can cause problems in relationships.

Experts Interviewed

In the video segment of this lesson, the following health professionals share their expertise to help you understand the material presented.

Robert A. Johnson, International Lecturer and Author

Toby Myers, Ed.D., Director, The PIVOT Project of Aid to Victims of Domestic Abuse, Houston, Texas, Lifetime Board Member, Texas Council on Family Violence

Video Focus Points

The following questions are designed to help you get the most from the video segment of this lesson. Review them before you watch the video. After viewing the video segment, write responses to reinforce what you have learned.

1. What are some of the important considerations in selecting a partner? What part do attraction, romance, and love play in a relationship?

2. Discuss characteristics important in intimate relationships.

3. What kinds of things are important in sustaining long-term intimate relationships?

4. How do problems of violence develop in relationships? What can be done to improve these relationships?

Individual Health Plan

This portion of the lesson is designed to enable you to apply the information you have learned to your own life situation and improve the quality of your life. You should do any exercise assigned, complete the journal portion of the plan, then put this portion of the health plan into practice in your life.

> Complete the Self-Assessment in your textbook, p. 176 If you have a significant other in your life, have that person complete it also. Compare and discuss your answers.

In your journal, write about those individuals with whom you have an intimate relationship. List the factors and characteristics that make the relationship intimate and special. List the characteristics that you bring to a relationship. List the characteristics that a potential partner must bring to a relationship for you to be interested in building a long-term relationship. If you and your significant other differ in many ways, develop some plans for how the two of you will work through the differences.

Enrichment Opportunities

These suggestions guide you if you want more information on this lesson, want to explore new ideas, or if your instructor requires it. If you are doing this section as a course requirement, consult with your instructor for specific guidelines or directions.

1. Interview some of your friends who are married, some who are single, and some who are cohabiting. Ask them about their thoughts on intimacy. Ask them about the characteristics of their relationships, what strengths they have, and what difficulties they encounter.

2. Visit or call an agency that deals with battered spouses and domestic violence. Ask what kinds of issues seem to lead to violence, what are typical outcomes, and other questions that you are concerned about.

Practice Test

After reading the assignment and watching the video, you should be able to answer the Practice Test questions. Tests also include essay questions that are similar to the Textbook Focus Points, the Video Focus Points, and the Objectives. When you have completed the Practice Test questions, turn to the Answer Key to score your answers.

1. Although intimate relationships change as people grow, the need for intimacy
   A. increases as one grows older.
   B. decreases as one grows older.
   C. becomes strongest during adolescence.
   D. remains strong at all ages.

2. The two essential qualities for any type of love are
   A. passion and attraction.
   B. caring and respect.
   C. intellect and emotion.
   D. curiosity and flexibility.

3. A single person is likely to experience the increased difficulty of
   A. fulfilling career demands.
   B. meeting emotional needs.
   C. generating sufficient discretionary income.
   D. maintaining a home.

4. No-fault divorce laws were established in order to
   A. make divorce more difficult.
   B. ease problems involved in getting a divorce.
   C. provide men greater custody rights than they once had.
   D. give women the right to collect alimony.

5. Factors that have been found to be related to the incidence of family violence include all of the following EXCEPT
   A. victims of abuse as children.
   B. single parents.
   C. low socioeconomic status.
   D. unemployment and poverty.

6. Common problems in intimate relationships LESS frequently include
   A. religion.
   B. divisions of labor.
   C. money.
   D. sex.

7. Sending flowers and taking the partner out to dinner exemplifies the part of the relationship that is termed
   A. attraction.
   B. romance.
   C. physical love.
   D. companionate love.

8. Important requirements for intimacy include all the following EXCEPT
   A. trust.
   B. openness.
   C. sex.
   D. deep caring.

9. Most people feel that the one most important factor in sustaining a long-term, intimate relationship is
   A. sexual compatibility.
   B. financial agreement.
   C. romance.
   D. communication.

10. The perpetrator of violence in a relationship is usually the one who is more
   A. right.
   B. intelligent.
   C. powerful.
   D. angry.

11. At the outset, most marriages are based on _____.

12. As women have become less economically dependent on their husbands, increase has occurred in rates of _____.

13. Social and environmental stressors are related to the incidence of domestic _____.

14. The initial, positive impression that an individual has of another is termed _____.

True or False
15. People who marry are least likely to match up with each other in compatibility of interests.

16. Cohabitation is a lifestyle of the young and restless.

17. Abused partners usually stay in abusive situations because they are misguided and emotionally unstable.

18. When partners in a relationship get to the point that they say, "we never fight," the relationship is very good.

19. Openness and honesty are important characteristics of successful intimate relationships.

20. Sustaining a successful long-term relationship involves surrendering one's individuality.

Answer Key

These are the correct answers with reference to the Learning Objectives, and to the source of the information: the Textbook Focus Points, Levy, *et al. Life and Health,* and the Video Focus Points. Page numbers are also given for the Textbook Focus Points. "KT" indicates questions with Key Terms defined.

Question	Answer	Learning Objective	Textbook Focus Point (page no.)	Video Focus Point
1.	D	8.1	1 (p. 170)	
2.	B	8.2	2 (p. 172)	
3.	B	8.2	3 (p. 175)	
4.	B	8.3	4 (p. 177)	
5.	B	8.3	5 (p. 186)	
6.	A	8.1	6 (p. 190)	
7.	B	8.2		1
8.	C	8.1		2
9.	D	8.1		3
10.	C	8.3		4
11.	romantic love	8.2	2 (p. 172)	KT
12.	divorce	8.3	4 (p. 177)	
13.	violence	8.3	5 (p. 186)	
14.	attraction	8.2		1
15.	F	8.2	2 (p. 173)	
16.	F	8.2	3 (p. 175)	
17.	F	8.3	5 (p. 187)	
18.	F	8.1	6 (p. 191)	
19.	T	8.1		2
20.	F	8.1		3

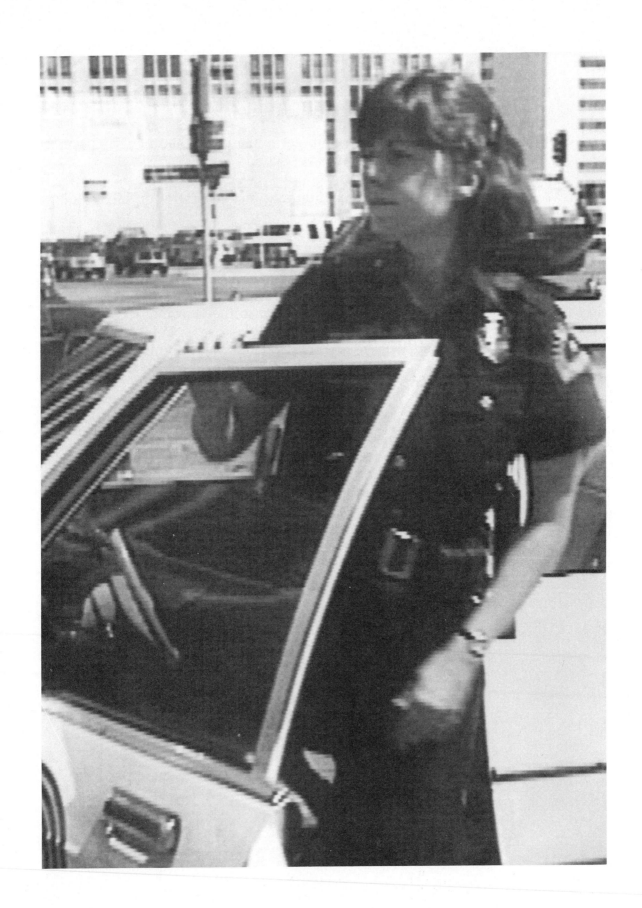

Lesson 9

Sexuality

But it is not only men who have accepted the patriarchal version of reality. Women also have been taught to idealize masculine values at the expense of the feminine side of life. Many women have spent their lives in a constant feeling of inferiority because they felt that to be feminine was 'second best.' Women have been trained that only masculine activities, thinking, power, and achieving have any real value. Thus Western woman finds herself in the same psychological dilemma as Western man: developing a one-sided, competitive mastery of the masculine qualities at the expense of her feminine side.

Robert A. Johnson in *We*

Overview

Of all the aspects of health, sex and sexuality are probably the most emotionally "charged" and subject to the most myths and misconceptions. We all think about, read about, and are constantly bombarded by the media with messages about sex and sexuality. In spite of this, we frequently are not very sure how we really feel about our own sexuality. Sometimes we even have feelings of guilt about it.

We are all sexual beings. Our gender development begins before we are born. After birth, society places certain expectations on us, depending on our sex. Though our fundamental sense of our maleness or femaleness is set by the time we are about three years old, the expression of our sexuality changes through our life. These expressions of our sexuality make us feel comfortable about ourselves or they can cause tension in our lives. If we have learned to feel comfortable about our sexuality, we will usually feel comfortable with who we are, and be able to enjoy an intimate sexual relationship. If we have learned to feel uncomfortable with our sexuality, we may have considerable difficulty.

Important to a healthy sexuality is an understanding of our sexual anatomy and physiology — in other words, how we work. Here, lack of clear understanding again creates more misconceptions and problems than almost any other aspect of sexuality. For some reason, we often feel more comfortable about any other part of our anatomy and physiology than we do about our sexual selves. If you have not done it already, learn about your sexuality now and enjoy it.

Now is also a good time to consider the difference between sex and sexuality. Sex, whether we are talking about gender or intercourse, is only a part of sexuality. Our sexuality encompasses who we are, and has even been said to be the "sum total of our personality." Responsible sexual behavior is an important part of that whole picture known as our sexuality. In a caring and supportive intimate relationship, sexual intercourse adds a very special dimension. If the relationship is demeaning or exploitive, the sexual part is also damaging.

Our sexuality is fundamental to our good health. Our decisions about sexual behavior need to help us develop and nurture relationships, rather than hurt or degrade them. If we make responsible decisions, communicate openly, and truly value the relationship, our sexuality will reflect the very best of human intimacy.

Learning Objectives

Goal: You should be able to discuss issues of human sexuality and responsible sexual expression.

Objectives: Upon completion of this lesson, you should be able to:

1. Discuss sexuality, attitudes toward sex, various forms of sexual expression, unacceptable sexual behavior, and responsible expression.

2. Describe sexual anatomy and physiology, the sexual response, and common sexual problems and dysfunctions.

Study Assignments

Pay careful attention to the following assignments. The chapter number may not be the same as the lesson number.

Textbook: Chapter 8, "Human Sexuality," pp. 196-223

Video: "Sexuality"

Key Terms

Watch for these terms and pay particular attention to what each one means, as you follow the textbook and video.

Gender	Ejaculation
Sexuality	Refractory period
Core gender identity	Circumcision
Erogenous zones	Masturbation
Urethra	Foreplay
Glans	Cunnilingus
Frenulum	Fellatio
Scrotum	Homosexuality
Epididymis	Heterosexuality
Perineum	Sexual dysfunction
Vulva	Premature ejaculation
Mons veneris	Retarded ejaculation
Labia	Impotence
Vagina	Secondary impotence
Hymen	Anorgasmia
Vasocongestion	Situational anorgasmia
Myotonia	Dyspareunia
Orgasm	

Textbook Focus Points

Before you read the textbook assignment, review the following points to help focus your thoughts. After you complete the assignment, write out your responses to reinforce what you have learned.

1. Discuss the basis of sexuality and attitudes toward sex and sexuality. How do most people first learn about sex and sexuality?

2. Describe the structures and functions of the male and female sexual anatomy.

3. Explain the physiology of the sexual response. Include some common misconceptions.

4. Discuss the various forms of sexual expression. Point out unacceptable sexual behavior.

5. Describe common sexual problems and sexual dysfunction. What are the goals of sex therapy?

6. Discuss the concept of responsible sexual expression.

Experts Interviewed

In the video segment of this lesson, the following health professionals share their expertise to help you understand the material presented.

Barbara S. Cambridge, Ph.D., Associate Professor of Obstetrics and Gynecology, The University of Texas Southwestern Medical Center, Dallas, Texas

Sue James, M.S., Clinical Supervisor, Dallas County Rape Crisis and Child Sexual Abuse Center, Dallas, Texas

Video Focus Points

The following questions are designed to help you get the most from the video segment of this lesson. Review them before you watch the video. After viewing the video segment, write responses to reinforce what you have learned.

1. How have attitudes about sex, sexuality, and gender roles changed in recent years?

2. What role does sex play in a relationship that is nurturing, caring, and sharing?

3. Explain the boundaries between sex that is nurturing and that which is unacceptable and demeaning. Include a discussion of rape as an act of violence.

Individual Health Plan

This portion of the lesson is designed to enable you to apply the information you have learned to your own life situation and improve the quality of your life. You should do any exercise assigned, complete the journal portion of the plan, then put this portion of the health plan into practice in your life.

In your journal, record your feelings about your own sexuality. Complete the self-assessment on pages 212-213 of your textbook. Using the insight gained from these activities, develop you own plans for responsible sexual expression. Be certain these plans fit you and are not what you think someone else expects of you.

Enrichment Opportunities

These suggestions guide you if you want more information on this lesson, want to explore new ideas, or if your instructor requires it. If you are doing this section as a course requirement, consult with your instructor for specific guidelines or directions.

1. Interview a sex therapist to learn more about sexual problems in relationships and their treatment.

2. Discuss the subject of sexuality with some of your close friends of both sexes. Compare and contrast the different ideas.

3. Find out how a rape crisis center operates, some of the problems suffered by rape victims, and some of the legal aspects of a rape investigation.

Practice Test

After reading the assignment and watching the video, you should be able to answer the Practice Test questions. Tests also include essay questions that are similar to the Textbook Focus Points, the Video Focus Points, and the Objectives. When you have completed the Practice Test questions, turn to the Answer Key to score your answers.

1. The fundamental sense of oneself as a male or female, which usually is established by age 3, is called one's
   A. genital sexual identity.
   B. core gender identity.
   C. sexual personality.
   D. sexuality.

2. Areas of the body that produce sexual arousal when stimulated are called
   A. erogenous zones.
   B. sensual zones.
   C. stimulant zones.
   D. erroneous zones.

3. The stage of sexual response in which the testicles swell from increased blood flow and the uterus elevates and moves back toward the spine is called
   A. orgasm.
   B. refractory.
   C. plateau.
   D. resolution.

4. Today, authorities agree that masturbation
   A. limits an individual's creativity.
   B. decreases an individual's problem-solving skills.
   C. provides a legitimate way of exploring the body.
   D. seems appropriate only for teenagers.

5. Impotence refers to
   A. male inability to attain an erection.
   B. male inability to produce orgasm in the female.
   C. ejaculation prior to penetration.
   D. ejaculation soon after penetration.

6. A negative aspect of the changing attitudes about sex and sexuality is the
   A. growth of the women's movement.
   B. perception of sexuality as a "closet" topic.
   C. exploitation of women and sexuality.
   D. development of a men's movement.

7. In a nurturing relationship, sex
   A. occurs at least once a week.
   B. plays a minor role.
   C. presents many problems.
   D. deepens the relationship.

8. During which of the following circumstances is sex always unacceptable?
   A. It is exploitive.
   B. It is not wanted by one partner.
   C. It is demeaning.
   D. All of the above

9. The head of the penis is called the _____.

10. Before ejaculation, the Cowper's glands secrete a small amount of fluid that cleanses the _____.

11. The urethra, penis, and prostate gland contract, forcing semen out of the tip of the penis during _____.

12. The inability of a woman to reach orgasm is called _____.

13. Coercing a person to engage in sexual intercourse when the person resists is considered _____.

True or False
14. There is a difference in sex and sexuality.

15. The labia is the canal-like structure that extends from the vulva to the internal sexual organs.

16. Women are often raped by men they know.

17. Responsible and healthy sexuality involves a consideration of the feelings and needs of others as well as one's own.

18. Attitudes about sex and sexuality have changed little through the years.

19. When a relationship is nurturing and caring, sex plays only a minor role.

20. The psychological effects of rape on the victim begin with extreme fear and extend to long-term feelings of lack of control and questioning oneself.

Answer Key

These are the correct answers with reference to the Learning Objectives, and to the source of the information: the Textbook Focus Points, Levy, *et al. Life and Health,* and the Video Focus Points. Page numbers are also given for the Textbook Focus Points. "KT" indicates questions with Key Terms defined.

Question	Answer	Learning Objective	Textbook Focus Point (page no.)		Video Focus Point
1.	B	9.1	1 (p. 198)	KT	
2.	A	9.2	2 (p. 202)	KT	
3.	C	9.2	3 (p. 206)		
4.	C	9.1	4 (p. 210)		
5.	A	9.2	5 (p. 217)	KT	
6.	C	9.1			1
7.	D	9.1			2
8.	D	9.1			3
9.	glans	9.2	2 (p. 203)	KT	
10.	urethra	9.2	2 (p. 204)		
11.	ejaculation	9.2	3 (p. 207)	KT	
12.	anorgasmia	9.2	5 (p. 219)	KT	
13	rape	9.1			3
14.	T	9.1	1 (p. 197)		
15.	F	9.2	2 (p. 204)	KT	
16.	T	9.1	4 (p. 214)		
17.	T	9.1	6 (p. 220)		
18.	F	9.1			1
19.	F	9.1			2
20.	T	9.1			3

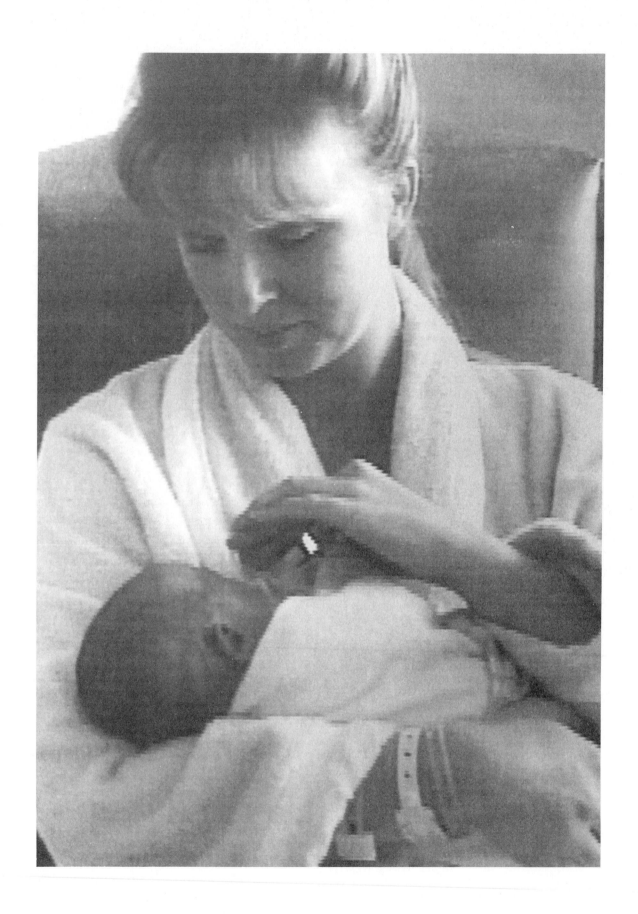

Lesson 10

Reproduction and Sexual Health

Birth is a metaphor for life. How we plan for it, how we experience it, how we feel about it afterward are all part of who we are.

Rahima Baldwin and Terra Palmarini, *Pregnant Feelings*

Overview

Many of us think of sexual intercourse as simply a part of an intimate relationship, and give little thought to its role in beginning a new life. Thus, sexual intercourse is intertwined with the most significant decision that we will ever make — the decision to have children. Never before in history have there ever been so many issues involving sexual health. For this reason, this lesson is particularly important. The decisions you make about your sexual activity will greatly influence your overall health.

Having intercourse without understanding the anatomy and physiology of reproduction, birth control options, and the process of pregnancy can be compared to taking a very hot sports car for a spin without learning to drive. Lack of knowledge and sexual irresponsibility frequently result in sexually transmitted diseases, problem pregnancies, unwanted children, and child abuse. Knowledge, understanding, and responsible behavior result in mature, caring relationships and nurtured children. There are also differing values concerning birth control. The important thing to consider is that sexual intercourse without some form of birth control amounts to a decision to have children.

There is nothing more remarkable than the growth of a single cell into a perfectly formed human infant. When you consider how many things can happen in the process of conception, the development of the embryo into a fetus, and the growth of the fetus during pregnancy, the remarkable becomes a true miracle. In spite of incredible progress in medicine and technology in treating problems of the fetus and newborn, the United States has a staggering number of infants suffering from the effects of parental substance abuse and other preventable problems. These babies are really the ones who are suffering from the neglect and abuse of their parents. Pregnancy is probably the most important time of our life to practice a healthy lifestyle, not only for ourself, but for the precious life that is to come.

If you have or plan to have a sexual relationship, it is imperative that you examine your sexual health behavior and values. This lesson is not about telling you **what** to think about birth control, abortion, and other sexual issues. It is about encouraging you **to** think, and make responsible sexual health decisions based on your own knowledge and values.

Learning Objectives

Goal: You should be able to explain the reproductive process, contraception, pregnancy, and childbirth.

Objectives: Upon completion of this lesson, you should be able to:

1. Describe the anatomy and physiology of reproduction, menstruation, and menopause.

2. Explain the various contraceptive methods, their effectiveness, advantages, and disadvantages.

3. Discuss pregnancy; including factors in planning a pregnancy, diagnosis and testing, problems, and health behaviors important to prenatal health.

4. Explain fetal development and childbirth.

Study Assignments

Pay careful attention to the following assignments. The chapter number may not be the same as the lesson number.

Textbook: Chapter 9, "Reproduction and Sexual Health," pp. 224-254

Video: "Reproduction and Sexual Health"

Key Terms

Watch for these terms and pay particular attention to what each one means, as you follow the textbook and video.

Ovum
Ovaries
Menarche
Ovulation
Fallopian tubes
Uterus
Cervix
Endometrium
Menstrual cycle
Menstruation
Premenstrual syndrome (PMS)
Menopause
Testes
Sperm
Spermatogenesis
Epididymis
Vas deferens
Seminal vesicles
Prostate gland
Semen (seminal fluid)
Ejaculatory ducts

Cowper's glands
Condom
Withdrawal
Oral contraceptives
Intrauterine device (IUD)
Diaphragm
Vasectomy
Tubal ligation
Amniocentesis
Chorionic villi sampling
Placenta
Prenatal
Umbilical cord
Amnion (amniotic sac)
Fetal Alcohol Syndrome
Toxemia
Spontaneous abortion
Abortion
Episiotomy
Cesarean section

Text Focus Points

Before you read the textbook assignment, review the following points to help focus your thoughts. After you complete the assignment, write out your responses to reinforce what you have learned.

1. Describe the anatomy and physiology of the female and male reproductive organs.

2. Explain the process of menstruation and menopause including psychological effects.

3. Discuss the various contraceptive methods, including their level of effectiveness, advantages, and disadvantages. Include contraceptives of the future.

4. What diseases might be avoided through genetic counseling? Describe tests for genetic disorders. Under what circumstances are amniocentesis or similar tests recommended to any pregnant woman?

5. Discuss the development of the fetus and the diagnosis and testing for pregnancy.

6. What are the health behaviors important to insuring prenatal health?

7. Discuss the common problems that can occur during pregnancy. Describe methods used for terminating a pregnancy.

8. Describe the childbirth process, including choices in childbirth methods.

Experts Interviewed

In the video segment of this lesson, the following medical and health professionals share their expertise to help you understand the material presented.

Timothy R.B. Johnson, M.D., Professor and Chair, Obstetrics and Gynecology, University of Michigan, Ann Arbor, Michigan

Carin Hanratty, R.N., P.N.P., Pediatric Coordinator for Drug Exposed Babies, Parkland Memorial Hospital, Dallas, Texas

Video Focus Points

The following questions are designed to help you get the most from the video segment of this lesson. Review them before you watch the video. After viewing the video segment, write responses to reinforce what you have learned.

1. How does the mother maintain health for herself and the developing child through pregnancy?

2. Describe the development of the fetus through the three trimesters of pregnancy. Include the changes taking place in the mother.

3. Describe the process of birth.

4. How do unhealthy lifestyle behaviors of the mother such as drug abuse affect the developing child?

Individual Health Plan

This portion of the lesson is designed to enable you to apply the information you have learned to your own life situation and improve the quality of your life. You should do any exercise assigned, complete the journal portion of the plan, then put this portion of the health plan into practice in your life.

> In your journal, write down your values and beliefs concerning sexual activity, birth control, and pregnancy. Writing them down helps clarify them for you. Now examine your sexual behavior. Does your behavior match your beliefs and values? Is it responsible in terms of what you have learned? If you are behaving responsibly in concert with your values, be comfortable with what you are doing. If not, develop a sexual health plan congruent with your values and what you have learned in this lesson.

Enrichment Opportunities

These suggestions guide you if you want more information on this lesson, want to explore new ideas, or if your instructor requires it. If you are doing this section as a course requirement, consult with your instructor for specific guidelines or directions.

1. Research the current abortion issues from the various points of view.

2. Visit the various types of childbirth facilities in your community. Compare and contrast them in terms of safety, competency of staff, comfort, and support for parents and baby.

Practice Test

After reading the assignment and watching the video, you should be able to answer the Practice Test questions. Tests also include essay questions that are similar to the Text Focus Points, the Video Focus Points, and the Objectives. When you have completed the Practice Test questions, turn to the Answer Key to score your answers.

1. Unripened ova are created in
   A. the first phase of the monthly menstrual cycle.
   B. a woman's ovaries at birth.
   C. a woman's ovaries after menarche.
   D. the uterus when sperm cells enter.

2. Menstruation is the
   A. preparation of the uterus for a fertilized ovum.
   B. release from the body of progesterone.
   C. sloughing off of the thickened uterine lining.
   D. monthly period during which ova are created.

3. What is the most effective contraceptive method?
   A. Condoms
   B. Rhythm
   C. Abstinence
   D. Vaginal sponge

4. Diseases that might be avoided through genetic counseling prior to pregnancy do NOT include
   A. sickle-cell anemia.
   B. hemophilia.
   C. cystic fibrosis.
   D. fetal alcohol syndrome.

5. The mass of tissue attached to the uterine lining and to the child, which provides nutrients and oxygen to the fetus and carries away fetal wastes is called the
   A. placenta.
   B. amniotic sac.
   C. zygote.
   D. embryo.

6. The LEAST hazardous substance for the developing fetus is
   A. alcohol.
   B. tobacco.
   C. caffeine.
   D. calcium.

7. Common problems associated with pregnancy that pose little threat to the health of the mother or fetus do NOT include
   A. morning sickness.
   B. constipation.
   C. toxemia.
   D. heartburn.

8. Normally, the first sign that true labor is about to begin is indicated by
   A. significant vaginal bleeding.
   B. draining of the amniotic fluid.
   C. contractions of the uterus.
   D. cervical dilation.

9. Healthy lifestyle behaviors for the pregnant woman do NOT include
   A. balanced diet.
   B. regular exercise.
   C. occasional glasses of wine.
   D. multivitamins.

10. During the second trimester of pregnancy, the fetus
    A. develops its heart.
    B. grows significantly in length.
    C. gains most of its weight.
    D. remains unrecognizable.

11. During the first stage of labor, the cervix
    A. dilates.
    B. contracts.
    C. remains the same.
    D. closes.

12. When the mother uses drugs during pregnancy, the baby is
    A. born overweight.
    B. born addicted.
    C. generally unaffected.
    D. stillborn.

13. The male reproductive cells are called _____.

14. A shallow rubber cup used to cover the cervix completely to prevent sperm from entering the uterus is called _____.

15. Care for a baby before birth is called _____.

16. The pregnancy is divided into thirds, each period called a
_____.

True or False

17. Latest research proves that premenstrual syndrome (PMS) is in the woman's imagination.

18. Parenthood and pregnancy require a significant amount of planning.

19. Because of danger to the developing fetus, exercise is discouraged for the pregnant woman.

20. Effects of drug abuse by the mother affect the baby in very dangerous ways.

Answer Key

These are the correct answers with reference to the Learning Objectives, and to the source of the information: the Textbook Focus Points, Levy, *et al. Life and Health,* and the Video Focus Points. Page numbers are also given for the Textbook Focus Points. "KT" indicates questions with Key Terms defined.

Question	Answer	Learning Objective	Textbook Focus Point (page no.)		Video Focus Point
1.	B	10.1	1 (p. 226)	KT	
2.	C	10.1	2 (p. 227)	KT	
3.	C	10.2	3 (p. 232)		
4.	D	10.3	4 (p. 241)		
5.	A	10.4	5 (p. 243)	KT	
6.	D	10.3	6 (p. 245)		
7.	C	10.3	7 (p. 246)	KT	
8.	B	10.4	8 (p. 250)		
9.	C	10.3			1
10.	B	10.4			2
11.	A	10.4			3
12.	B	10.3			4
13.	sperm	10.1	1 (p. 230)	KT	
14.	diaphragm	10.2	3 (p. 236)	KT	
15.	prenatal care	10.4	5 (p. 243)		
16.	trimester	10.4			2
17.	F	10.1	2 (pp. 228-229)		
18.	T	10.3	4 (p. 241)		
19.	F	10.3			1
20.	T	10.3			4

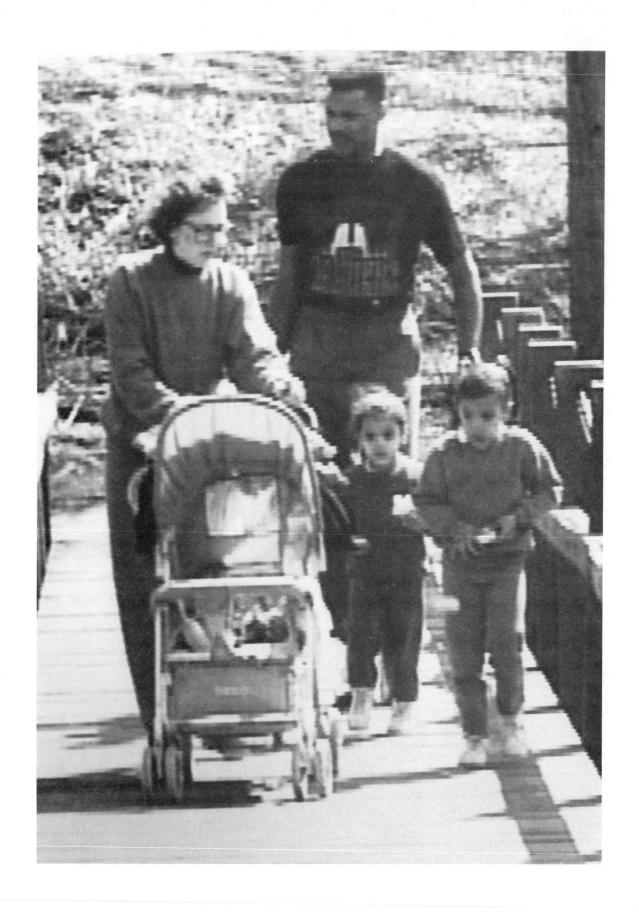

Lesson 11

Parenting

There are only two lasting bequests that we can hope to give our children. One of these is roots; the other, wings.

Hodding Carter

Overview

Though many people think of marriage as the greatest commitment that we make in our lives, it is not. Parenthood is that supreme commitment. Children are forever. We may divorce our spouse, but we do not divorce our children. Many of us envision that darling little baby enriching our lives (and they certainly do), but give less thought to the responsibility that we take on when we become parents. The decision to become a parent means that we will protect, nurture, feed, clothe, shelter, and love that child 24 hours a day, 365 days a year. We never stop being parents. For most of us, it is a joyful responsibility, although a big one. Because it is important that we are ready to take responsibility for children, we must make clear decisions about our sexual behavior. If we have made these decisions and have realistic expectations of parenthood, we are ready to cope with the difficulties and to enjoy the unique experiences we share with our children.

While we have impact on our children's lives in many ways, the primary influence we have is on their health at birth and throughout their growth and development. As the five dimensions of health are important to us, they are important to our children. Our parenting has a significant effect on our children's physical, emotional, intellectual, social, and spiritual development. Planning for this begins before the child is conceived, and continues on. Responsibility for insuring that the child has a lifestyle that develops the five dimensions cannot be ignored or delegated. It belongs to us as parents.

Unfortunately, the antithesis of the healthy functioning family has become a very real problem in the United States today. Family violence and child abuse are at epidemic proportions. Reasons for this are many, but a

Parenting

common thread is stress within the family. In our roles as individuals, spouses, and parents, we will experience stress. It is important to the well-being of our children and ourselves, that we learn healthy ways of coping and parenting. It is up to us to make certain that our children are not raised in an atmosphere of violence.

While all of this may sound very one-sided, we get much from our children. It has been said that children are our mirror, and this is at least partially true. Children respond and flourish with good parenting. They give us a sense of accomplishment and purpose, and enrich the quality of our life immensely. For all the difficulties and demands, most people cherish the parental experience above all else.

Learning Objectives

Goal: You should be able to explain the role and responsibilities of parenthood in the healthy growth and development of the child.

Objectives: Upon completion of this lesson, you should be able to:

1. Describe parental responsibilities from the decision to have a child through the role in developing the five dimensions of health in the child.

2. Explain the parents' role in caring for the child, and the child's contribution to the parent-child relationship.

3. Discuss the problems in child rearing including child abuse, its risk factors, and what to do if you suspect child abuse.

Study Assignments

Pay careful attention to the following assignments. The chapter number may not be the same as the lesson number.

Textbook: Chapter 7, "Marriage, Family, and Other Intimate Relationships," pp. 178-187

Video: "Parenting"

Key Terms

There are no new Key Terms in this lesson.

Text Focus Points

Before you read the textbook assignment, review the following points to help focus your thoughts. After you complete the assignment, write out your responses to reinforce what you have learned.

1. Discuss the various aspects of the decision to have a child. Include healthy and unhealthy reasons, and distinguish between the two.

2. Describe the parental role in developing the five dimensions of health — physical, emotional, intellectual, social, and spiritual — for the child.

3. What contribution does the child bring to the parent-child relationship?

4. Explain the mother's and father's role in caring for the child in today's society. Include the challenges of being a single parent. What are some of the other child care possibilities?

5. Discuss the problems of child rearing, including child abuse. Include the risk factors and what one should do if child abuse is suspected.

Experts Interviewed

In the video segment of this lesson, the following medical and health professionals share their expertise to help you understand the material presented.

Alvin F. Poussaint, M.D., Senior Associate of Psychiatry, Judge Baker Children's Center, Boston, Massachusetts

John R. Shepperd, Investigator, Criminal District Attorney's Office, Dallas County, Texas

---

Video Focus Points

The following questions are designed to help you get the most from the video segment of this lesson. Review them before you watch the video. After viewing the video segment, write responses to reinforce what you have learned.

1. In what ways has the role of parenthood changed through recent years?

2. Explain the ways in which parents help their children grow in the five dimensions, physical, emotional, intellectual, social, and spiritual.

3. Describe some of the special challenges that are faced by single parents.

4. Discuss the scope of child abuse in the United States, the affects of abuse on children's health, and things that lower the risk of child abuse.

Individual Health Plan

This portion of the lesson is designed to enable you to apply the information you have learned to your own life situation and improve the quality of your life. You should do any exercise assigned, complete the journal portion of the plan, then put this portion of the health plan into practice in your life.

In your journal, make a list of your own reasons for having and for not having a child at this time. (Do this even if you have children.) Also list the adjustments you would have to make in your life if you did have a child at this time. Include child care planning if both parents work or if yours is a single parent family. How would you adjust your budget to accommodate a child. Write a synopsis of what you found. Are you ready??

Enrichment Opportunities

These suggestions guide you if you want more information on this lesson, want to explore new ideas, or if your instructor requires it. If you are doing this section as a course requirement, consult with your instructor for specific guidelines or directions.

1. If you do not have children, interview the parents of children of various ages, concerning the positive experiences and difficulties of parenting.

2. Visit different types of child care facilities. Find out about their programs, costs, licensing, etc.

Practice Test

After reading the assignment and watching the video, you should be able to answer the Practice Test questions. Tests also include essay questions that are similar to the Text Focus Points, the Video Focus Points, and the Objectives. When you have completed the Practice Test questions, turn to the Answer Key to score your answers.

1. Which of the following is referred to as the ultimate responsibility and supreme commitment?
   A. Marriage
   B. Cohabitation
   C. Parenthood
   D. Dual career marriage

2. Offering choices to very young children will contribute to their
   A. physical development.
   B. emotional development.
   C. intellectual development.
   D. spiritual development.

3. Children first learn discipline from
   A. schools.
   B. churches.
   C. peers and older children.
   D. parents.

---

4. An important contribution of the child in the parent-child relationship is
   A. positive effect on the parents' psychological well-being.
   B. need for parents to establish order and rules.
   C. provision of care for parents in ill health.
   D. drain on the parents' financial resources.

5. Which of the following phrases best describes a father's contributions to a child's care?
   A. Energetic physical play.
   B. Quiet and loving nurturing.
   C. Distant and detached concern.
   D. Controlled teaching of verbal skills.

6. Individuals who were victims of abuse and violence as children are more likely than others are to become
   A. divorced.
   B. abusive adults.
   C. remarried.
   D. permissive parents.

7. Risk factors for a child being abused include all the following EXCEPT
   A. parental alcohol use.
   B. childhood health and developmental problems.
   C. discouragement of corporal punishment.
   D. parental stress.

8. Changes in the parenting role through the years do NOT include increase in
   A. single parents.
   B. importance of nurturing.
   C. involvement of the father.
   D. child abuse.

9. The most critical years in the development of the child are from
   A. birth to 5 years.
   B. 5 to 10 years.
   C. 8 to 12 years.
   D. 12 to 18 years.

10. The single parent most often feels the pressure of
    A. having too little money.
    B. being alone in caring for the child.
    C. feeling loneliness for the spouse.
    D. not wanting the child.

11. Child abuse occurs among
    A. lower socioeconomic groups only.
    B. all segments of society.
    C. mostly single parents.
    D. some ethnic groups more than others.

12. The ultimate responsibility that a couple can assume is
    _____.

13. According to Erik Erikson, parents, who convey a sense of relaxation and enjoyment, can help a child develop basic
    _____.

14. Parents need to make a child's environment as safe as possible in order to prevent accidents that might restrict the child's _____ development.

15. The most difficult form of child abuse to recognize is
    _____.

True or False
16. The passiveness of young infants contributes little to parent-child relationships.

17. The role of the mother has changed dramatically in some ways and has remained the same in others.

18. Joblessness, divorce, and poverty place great pressure on parents but are of little concern to children.

19. Children of single parents usually receive less nurturing than those in two-parent homes.

20. Support systems such as grandparents and other relatives decrease the risk for child abuse.

Answer Key

These are the correct answers with reference to the Learning Objectives, and to the source of the information: the Textbook Focus Points, Levy, *et al. Life and Health,* and the Video Focus Points. Page numbers are also given for the Textbook Focus Points. "KT" indicates questions with Key Terms defined.

Question	Answer	Learning Objective	Textbook Focus Point (page no.)	Video Focus Point
1.	C	11.1	1 (p. 178)	
2.	C	11.1	2 (p. 181)	
3.	D	11.1	2 (p. 181)	
4.	A	11.2	3 (pp. 181-182)	
5.	A	11.2	4 (p. 183)	
6.	B	11.3	5 (p. 186)	
7.	C	11.3	5 (p. 187)	
8.	B	11.2		1
9.	A	11.1		2
10.	B	11.2		3
11.	B	11.3		4
12.	parenthood	11.1	1 (p. 178)	
13.	trust	11.1	2 (p. 180)	
14.	physical	11.1	2 (p. 180)	
15.	emotional	11.3		4
16.	F	11.2	3 (p. 181)	
17.	T	11.2	4 (p. 182)	
18.	F	11.2		1
19.	F	11.2		3
20.	T	11.3		4

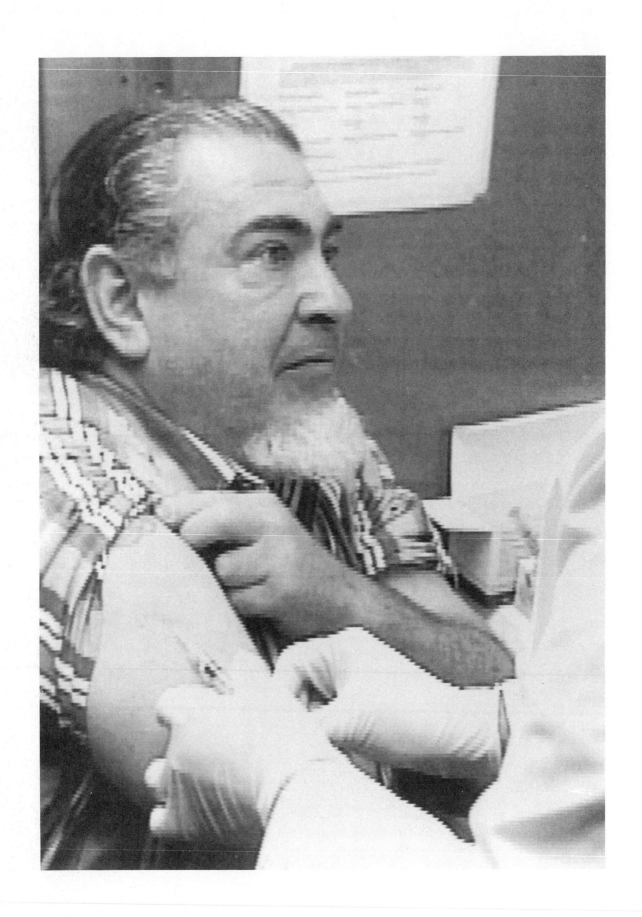

Lesson 12

Communicable Diseases

... I think the nuts and bolts that we have, the vaccines, the antibiotics, and the public health measures that limit exposure; that's where we're going to control infectious disease.

John Bartlett, M.D.

Overview

Disease has been a part of our lives since the dawn of history. Though the causes of many of the great epidemics of the past have been eradicated or brought under control, new diseases are constantly appearing: toxic shock syndrome, Lyme disease, AIDS. Old diseases thought to be under control reappear as threats when conditions change: tuberculosis. Some seem to have always been with us: colds, flu. Our lifestyle, travel, and the progress of medical science all have had a part in changing the patterns of the diseases that threaten us. Clearly the only constant is that, though their appearance may change, diseases remain a part of our lives now, and probably will in the foreseeable future.

Because we will be studying various types of disease throughout this course, it is important to understand the different classifications: acute, chronic, infectious, noninfectious, communicable, and noncommunicable. This lesson focuses on the infectious, communicable diseases. To use a simple term, these are diseases that you can "catch." The significance of these communicable diseases is seen many times through history. The "Black Plague" ravaged Europe in the Middle Ages. Groups of native people were wiped out by diseases caught from explorers. The extreme caution of NASA scientists during the first landing on the moon insured that we did not infect that environment with our organisms and that the mission did not bring any foreign organisms back to earth.

There are several useful models that scientists use to explain how people contract disease. As our textbook states, the agent-host-environment model demonstrates the multiplicity of factors that are involved in the onset of disease in the individual. The keys are in the interrelationships of the agent (disease-causing organisms), the host (characteristics of individuals that make them susceptible to the disease), and the environment (extrinsic biological, social, and physical factors that influence the probability of developing an infection).

It is important for us to understand the agents of infection, the ways in which our bodies fight infection, and ways to enhance our resistance to disease. If we practice good health habits based on an understanding of these principles, we will certainly add to our overall health and well-being.

Learning Objectives

Goal: You should be able to analyze the nature and patterns of disease, how diseases are contracted, the various agents of infection, the ways in which the body fights disease, and how to enhance resistance to infectious, communicable disease.

Objectives: Upon completion of this lesson, you should be able to:

1. Explain the nature of infectious disease, and how lifestyle, travel, and medical progress are related to changing patterns of disease.

2. Discuss the various organisms that cause disease, and the body's defenses against disease.

Study Assignments

Pay careful attention to the following assignments. The chapter number may not be the same as the lesson number.

Textbook: Chapter 10, "Communicable Diseases", pp. 257-274

Video: "Communicable Diseases"

Key Terms

Watch for these terms and pay particular attention to what each one means, as you follow the textbook and video.

Communicable disease	Virus
Noncommunicable disease	Rickettsiae
Infectious disease	Vector
Infection	Fungi
Agent factor	Prion
Host factor	Inflammation
Environmental factor	Inflammatory response
Incubation period	Phagocytes
Prodrome period	Abscess
Clinical disease	Immunity
Decline stage	Lymphocytes: B cells/T cells
Convalescence	Antibodies
Carrier	Antigens
Endogenous	Vaccine
Exogenous	Active immunity
Pathogen	Passive immunity
Bacterium (bacteria)	

Text Focus Points

Before you read the textbook assignment, review the following points to help focus your thoughts. After you complete the assignment, write out your responses to reinforce what you have learned.

1. How are lifestyle, travel, and medical progress related to the changing patterns of disease?

2. Explain the nature of infectious disease. Include the agent-host-environment factors, and the course of infectious disease.

3. Describe bacteria, viruses, rickettsiae, fungi, and prions and identify some of the diseases that they each cause.

4. Describe the body's defenses against infectious disease. Include the role of vaccines.

Experts Interviewed

In the video segment of this lesson, the following medical and health professionals share their expertise to help you understand the material presented.

John G. Bartlett, M.D., Chair, Department of Infectious Diseases, The Johns Hopkins University School of Medicine, Baltimore, Maryland

Ted L. Brown, M.S., Environmental Specialist, New Mexico Environmental Department, Santa Fe, New Mexico

Charles P. Felton, M.D., Chief, Division of Pulmonary Medicine, The Harlem Hospital Center, New York City, New York

Pam Reynolds, M.S. Environmental Specialist. New Mexico Environmmental Department, Santa Fe, New Mexico

Video Focus Point

The following questions are designed to help you get the most from the video segment of this lesson. Review them before you watch the video. After viewing the video segment, write responses to reinforce what you have learned.

1. How does the agent-host-environment model explain the spread of communicable disease?

2. How does infectious/communicable disease differ from other forms of disease?

3. How do changes in lifestyles, social conditions, and other factors change the incidence of and potential for communicable disease? Using tuberculosis as an example, explain how these factors change the potential for transmission of the disease.

4. Describe the three lines of defense the body has against communicable disease.

5. What control does the individual have over communicable disease?

Individual Health Plan

This portion of the lesson is designed to enable you to apply the information you have learned to your own life situation and improve the quality of your life. You should do any exercise assigned, complete the journal portion of the plan, then put this portion of the health plan into practice in your life.

Complete the self-assessment, "What is Your Attitude toward Sickness?" on page 261 of the text.

In your journal, using the knowledge you have gained in this lesson, write a paragraph discussing health habits that you practice thato decrease or increase your risk of contracting an infectious disease. Evaluate your lifestyle and make appropriate changes.

Enrichment Opportunities

These suggestions guide you if you want more information on this lesson, want to explore new ideas, or if your instructor requires it. If you are doing this section as a course requirement, consult with your instructor for specific guidelines or directions.

1. Explore the resurgence of tuberculosis as a public health threat by interviewing a health professional who works with patients who have the disease.

2. Interview a pediatric health professional and ask about the importance of childhood immunization.

3. Contact a health department official and discuss measures being taken in your community to prevent the spread of disease.

Practice Test

After reading the assignment and watching the video, you should be able to answer the Practice Test questions. Tests also include essay questions that are similar to the Text Focus Points, the Video Focus Points, and the Objectives. When you have completed the Practice Test questions, turn to the Answer Key to score your answers.

1. Patterns of disease have NOT been influenced by changing trends in
   A. work.
   B. diet.
   C. activity levels.
   D. microorganisms.

2. Which of the following is NOT an agent factor?
   A. Bacterium
   B. Fungus
   C. Rickettsia
   D. Immunity

3. The first stage of an infectious disease, when organisms invade and multiply in the host, is the
   A. clinical period.
   B. incubation period.
   C. prodrome period.
   D. decline period.

4. The primary differences between exogenous and endogenous microorganisms is residence inside or outside
   A. incubation.
   B. cells.
   C. hosts.
   D. bacteria.

5. Colds, flu, hepatitis, and mononucleosis are caused by
   A. viruses.
   B. bacteria.
   C. prions.
   D. fungi.

6. The group of mechanisms that helps protect the body against specific diseases is known as
   A. immunity.
   B. vaccine.
   C. interferon.
   D. antigen.

7. General health of the individual which contributes to vulnerability to a disease like tuberculosis is a condition of the
   A. environment.
   B. host.
   C. agent.
   D. bacteria.

8. Communicable diseases are caused by all the following EXCEPT
   A. bacteria.
   B. carcinogens.
   C. viruses.
   D. fungi.

9. The body's three lines of defense against disease include all the following EXCEPT
   A. antibiotics.
   B. skin and mucus membranes.
   C. immunity.
   D. inflammatory response.

10. A disease that cannot be spread from one person to another is _____.

11. The most plentiful microorganisms endogenous to humans are the various kinds of _____.

12. Irritant or foreign matter, whether a relatively large physical object, a chemical substance, or a microorganism, can be warded off by the _____ response.

13. Health habits that increase the potential for disease are factors relating to the _____.

14. The outside means by which the body's immunity can be increased is termed _____.

True or False

15. More frequent travelling by Americans has had no effect on the incidence of various diseases in the United States.

16. Air and water quality are examples of agent factors in the illness process.

17. Though permanent disability is unusual, symptoms of infectious mononucleosis may persist for months.

18. The skin and mucous membranes are the body's second line of defense.

19. Tuberculosis is a good example of a disease that has had a recurrence because of changes in factors related to the agent, hosts, and environments.

20. In contrast to many other diseases, the individual has very little control over the spread of communicable disease.

Answer Key

These are the correct answers with reference to the Learning Objectives, and to the source of the information: the Textbook Focus Points, Levy, *et al. Life and Health,* and the Video Focus Points. Page numbers are also given for the Textbook Focus Points. KT indicates questions with Key Terms defined.

Question	Answer	Learning Objective	Textbook Focus Point (page no.)		Video Focus Point
1.	D	12.1	1 (p. 258)		
2.	D	12.1	2 (p. 261)		
3.	B	12.1	2 (p. 262)	KT	
4.	C	12.2	3 (p. 262)		
5.	A	12.2	3 (pp. 265-267)		
6.	A	12.2	4 (p. 269)	KT	
7.	B	12.1			1
8.	B	12.1			2
9.	A	12.2			4
10.	noncommunicable	12.1	2 (p. 257)	KT	
11.	bacteria	12.2	3 (p. 263)	KT	
12.	inflammatory	12.2	4 (p. 269)	KT	
13.	host	12.1			1
14.	immunization		12..2		4
15.	F	12.1	1 (p. 259)		
16.	F	12.1	2 (p. 262)		
17.	T	12.2	3 (p. 267)		
18.	F	12.2	4 (p. 268)		
19.	T	12.1			3
20.	F	12.1			5

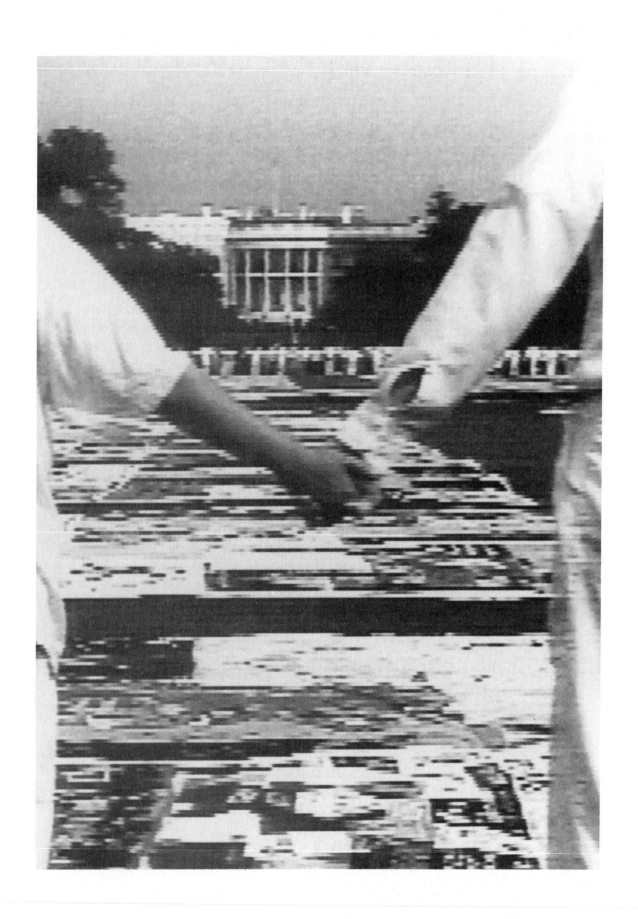

Lesson 13

AIDS and Sexually Transmitted Diseases

America is in great danger — not of catching AIDS — but of losing its humanity.....In all history there has never been a cure for that.

Belinda Mason

Overview

While most of the communicable diseases are on the decline, or at least under control, incidence of sexually transmitted diseases, including AIDS, is rising at an alarming rate. The reasons for this increase are many. The most important step in the solution, **prevention**, is the responsibility of all of us.

Though AIDS is receiving most of the attention at the present time, we cannot ignore the other sexually transmitted diseases (STDs), most of which have been around for a long time. We all know the severity of AIDS, but many of us overlook the severe and lasting effects the other STDs can have, such as sterility, abnormal pregnancy, and increased risk of cancer. Most STDs are caused by bacteria or viruses. Those caused by bacteria can usually be cured with antibiotics. Those caused by viruses cannot be cured because we have no cure for viral infections. Treatment is aimed at controlling the symptoms and preventing the spread of the disease to other people.

AIDS has received great attention, and those who have it are frequently ostracized and degraded. The truth is that AIDS is a disease, and the people who have it are entitled to our care and concern, just as those with any serious disease. Once thought to be a disease confined to homosexual people and intravenous drug users, now AIDS is understood to be a threat to almost everyone. We also know that the risk increases with the number of sexual partners. Because AIDS is a killer disease, with no cure at this time, **prevention** is the only answer.

While a few are exposed to AIDS and other sexually transmitted diseases through no action of their own, most are exposed through unprotected sexual intercourse, and in the case of AIDS, through the use of contaminated needles in intravenous drug use. This fact leads us back to the concept of gaining knowledge and being responsible for our own health behavior. The only completely "safe" sex is abstinence. Other than abstinence, using condoms and keeping to a monogamous relationship with a non-infected partner are the preventive measures we can take. In the case of AIDS, avoidance of exposure with contaminated intravenous drug paraphernalia is critical.

At the other end of the spectrum, we should not succumb to the hysteria of AIDS "phobia." Knowledge and understanding are crucial. Unless a cure is found very soon, all of us are going to be affected in some way by this epidemic. We must be a part of the solution to the problems of people with AIDS, rather than being part of the problem. Most important of all, we must take an active role in the **prevention** of the disease through our own responsible behavior.

Learning Objectives

Goal: You should be able to explain AIDS and other sexually transmitted diseases, and to describe responsible sexual behavior that prevents the spread of sexually transmitted diseases.

Objectives: Upon completion of this lesson, you should be able to:

1. Describe the various sexually transmitted diseases including AIDS, the patterns, their risks, symptoms, treatment, preventive measures, and implications for the future.

2. Discuss the impact of AIDS on the lives of the patient and family members.

Study Assignments

Pay careful attention to the following assignments. The chapter number may not be the same as the lesson number.

Textbook: Chapter 10, "Communicable Diseases," pp. 275-285

Video: "AIDS and Sexually Transmitted Diseases"

Key Terms

There are no new Key Terms for this lesson.

Text Focus Points

Before you read the textbook assignment, review the following points to help focus your thoughts. After you complete the assignment, write out your responses to reinforce what you have learned.

1. What are the trends in terms of the incidence of STDs in the United States? Describe the common sexually transmitted diseases, their risks, symptoms, and treatments. Describe the symptoms and treatment that can occur at each stage of syphilis.

2. Discuss AIDS in terms of the incidences, causative agents, modes of transmission, preventive measures, and treatment options.

3. What are the implications for the future in view of the politics of AIDS?

Experts Interviewed

In the video segment of this lesson, the following medical professionals share their expertise to help you understand the material presented.

Elisabeth Kübler-Ross, M.D., President, Elisabeth Kübler-Ross Center, Head Waters, Virginia

Jonathan M. Mann, M.D., M.P.H., Francois Xavier Bagnoud Professor of Health and Human Rights, Harvard School of Public Health, Boston, Massachusetts

L. Laurie Scott, M.D., Fellow, Maternal-Fetal Medicine, The University of Texas Southwestern Medical Center, Dallas, Texas

Video Focus Points

The following questions are designed to help you get the most from the video segment of this lesson. Review them before you watch the video. After viewing the video segment, write responses to reinforce what you have learned.

1. How widespread and of what significance is the problem of HIV, AIDS, and other sexually transmitted diseases?

2. Describe some of the most common sexually transmitted diseases other than HIV and AIDS.

3. Identify the primary modes of transmission of HIV. Describe the impact on the patient and family, and discuss prevention.

Individual Health Plan

This portion of the lesson is designed to enable you to apply the information you have learned to your own life situation and improve the quality of your life. You should do any exercise assigned, complete the journal portion of the plan, then put this portion of the health plan into practice in your life.

> Using the knowledge you have gained in this lesson, evaluate your own risk of contracting a sexually transmitted disease. In your journal, comment on any new or different information you have gained from this lesson. If it has caused any decision to change your behavior, comment on why it changed your beliefs. How have your views on AIDS changed or not changed?

Enrichment Opportunities

These suggestions guide you if you want more information on this lesson, want to explore new ideas, or if your instructor requires it. If you are doing this section as a course requirement, consult with your instructor for specific guidelines or directions.

1. Interview someone who works in an AIDS treatment or counseling center and find out what problems AIDS patients face.

2. Consider serving as a volunteer is some agency that serve AIDS patients.

Practice Test

After reading the assignment and watching the video, you should be able to answer the Practice Test questions. Tests also include essay questions that are similar to the Text Focus Points, the Video Focus Points, and the Objectives. When you have completed the Practice Test questions, turn to the Answer Key to score your answers.

1. Herpes genitalis is NOT
   A. associated with cancer of the cervix.
   B. threatening to the unborn child.
   C. prevalent throughout the U.S.
   D. responsive to antibiotics.

2. Syphilis is caused by a spiral shaped bacterium called a
   A. staphylococcus.
   B. spirochete.
   C. condyloma.
   D. trichomonas.

3. If untreated, what disease frequently leads to pelvic inflammatory disease, a painful condition that can cause sterility?
   A. Syphilis
   B. Condyloma
   C. Gonorrhea
   D. Herpes

4. In most cases the initial symptoms of HIV infection resemble those of
   A. herpes.
   B. cancer.
   C. condyloma.
   D. mononucleosis.

5. AIDS is described as the most severe form of
   A. cancer.
   B. HIV infection.
   C. yeast infection.
   D. syphilis.

6. Precautions for prevention of the spread of AIDS do NOT include
   A. limiting number of sexual partners.
   B. using condoms and other physical barriers during sexual activity.
   C. avoiding drug use, particularly intravenous injection.
   D. assuming that there is no threat.

7. Political issues related to AIDS do NOT include
   A. discrimination against AIDS patients.
   B. money to treat AIDS.
   C. effect on health insurance and medical care.
   D. practicing abstinence

8. One of the most disturbing things about AIDS is that it
   A. presents a problem in the U.S.
   B. affects primarily target groups.
   C. exists as a global problem.
   D. occurs primarily in third world countries.

9. A common viral, sexually transmitted disease that causes blisterlike sores around the genitalia and is very dangerous to the infant at birth is
   A. gonorrhea.
   B. genital herpes.
   C. chlamydia.
   D. HIV.

10. Prevention of AIDS includes all the following EXCEPT
    A. using condoms.
    B. avoiding IV drug use.
    C. taking preventive medication.
    D. limiting sexual partners.

11. The very commonly diagnosed, sexually transmitted disease characterized by warts in the genital area is known as genital warts or _____.

True or False

12. Sexually transmitted diseases are always viral in origin.

13. Syphilis is most contagious during the second stage yet causes the most damage to the individual in the tertiary stage.

14. If the sexual partner of an individual with chlamydia is asymptomatic, treatment of the partner is unnecessary.

15. AIDS is a disease of homosexual men.

16. Condoms or other physical barriers should be used even if the woman is already using oral contraceptives.

17. AZT is the only known cure for AIDS.

18. AIDS is the only really serious, sexually transmitted disease.

19. Chlamydia is a widely occurring, sexually transmitted disease affecting only women

20. Virtually everyone is affected in one way or another by the spread of AIDS.

Answer Key

These are the correct answers with reference to the Learning Objectives, and to the source of the information: the Textbook Focus Points, Levy, *et al. Life and Health,* and the Video Focus Points. Page numbers are also given for the Textbook Focus Points. "KT" indicates questions with Key Terms defined.

Question	Answer	Learning Objective	Textbook Focus Point (page no.)	Video Focus Point
1.	D	13.1	1 (pp. 276-277)	
2.	B	13.1	1 (p. 277)	
3.	C	13.1	1 (p. 278)	
4.	D	13.1	2 (p. 279)	
5.	B	13.1	2 (p. 280)	
6.	D	13.1	2 (pp. 280-281)	
7.	D	13.1	3 (p. 283)	
8.	C	13.1		1
9.	B	13.1		2
10.	C	13.1, 13.2		3
11.	condyloma	13.1		2
12.	F	13.1	1 (p. 276)	
13.	T	13.1	1 (pp. 277-278)	
14.	F	13.1	1 (p. 279)	
15.	F	13.1	2 (p. 279)	
16.	T	13.1	2 (p. 280)	
17.	F	13.1	2 (pp. 282-283)	
18.	F	13.1		1
19.	F	13.1		2
20.	T	13.1, 13.2		3

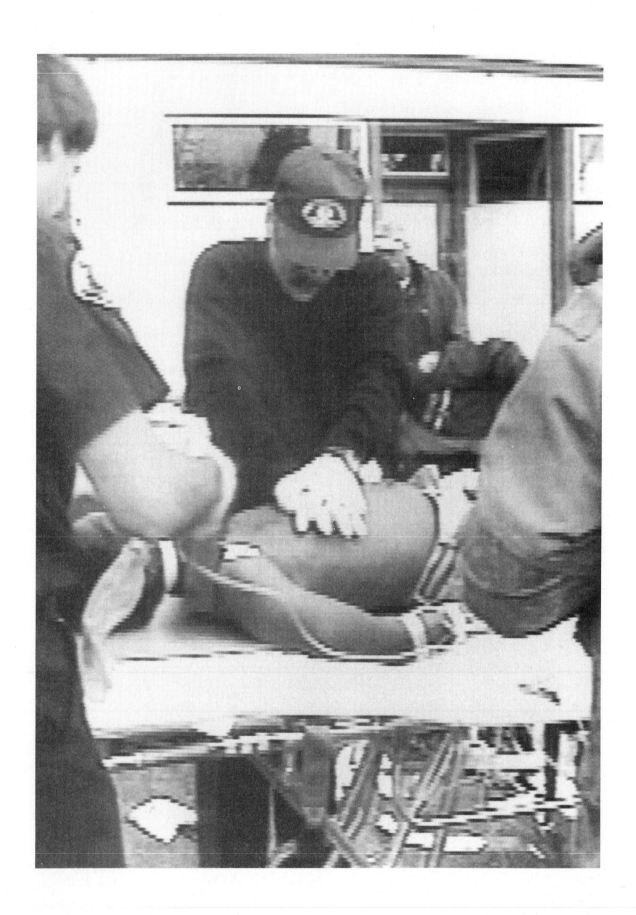

Lesson 14

Cardiovascular Disease

I was lying there on the table and they were taking my blood pressure and in the course of doing that, something profoundly occurred and I began to slip away. It was clear to me . . . there was a lightness, an unexpected lightness. I said to a person over me, I'm gonna die . . . .

Charles Wolfe, describing his heart attack

Overview

If you read newspaper obituaries, often you will see the expression, "died suddenly," referring to people who die of heart attacks. If we really think about this, we realize that this usually is not an accurate description of what happened. Cardiovascular disease usually is not sudden at all. It develops slowly and insidiously for many years, and is only sudden when it manifests itself as a full-blown heart attack. The process has been developing for a long time, since our early years, we just did not know it. For this reason, knowledge about cardiovascular disease and its prevention is crucial to our health.

In order to understand the cardiovascular diseases, it is important to understand something about the anatomy and physiology of the heart and circulatory system. Remember the heart is a pump sending the blood to the various organs. The blood vessels form the pipelines that carry the blood. Arteries carry blood (usually oxygenated) away from the heart, and veins carry deoxygenated blood back to the heart. The exception to this is the pulmonary circulation. The pulmonary arteries carry deoxygenated blood to the lungs, where it is oxygenated before being returned to the heart via the pulmonary veins. Understanding this will help you understand what can happen when the vessels become narrowed by disease, or when the heart is not pumping as effectively as it should.

Some of the most common and most important cardiovascular diseases are hypertension (high blood pressure), atherosclerosis, stroke, and myocardial infarction (heart attack). Yet, we can effectively lower our risk of these same diseases through lifestyle modification. The major risk factors for these diseases are smoking; obesity; a high fat, high salt diet; high blood cholesterol levels; lack of exercise; a family history of disease; and high blood pressure.

Because most of these cardiovascular conditions are relatively silent until they become quite far advanced, it is very important to pay attention if any of the danger signs appear. You should have your blood pressure checked on a regular basis. Any chest pain, shortness of breath, dizziness, indigestion, or heartburn should be evaluated by a physician. Too often we find that people deny the symptoms of cardiovascular disease until it is too late. If a person is having a heart attack, there is no time for delay. Time is critical to survival. Even if you "really don't" think this possibly could be a heart attack, it is essential to have it checked out.

Learning Objectives

Goal: You should be able to explain the cardiovascular diseases, the development of the diseases over time, and the risk factors associated with these diseases.

Objectives: Upon completion of this lesson, you should be able to:

1. Describe the anatomy and physiology of the heart and circulatory system, and explain hypertension and atherosclerosis as diseases and as causes of cardiovascular disease.

2. Discuss the following major cardiovascular diseases: heart attack, stroke, arrythmias, rheumatic heart disease, congenital heart defects, and congestive heart failure.

Study Assignments

Pay careful attention to the following assignments. The chapter number may not be the same as the lesson number.

Textbook: Chapter 11, "Cardiovascular Health and Disease," pp. 287-301, 303-305

Video: "Cardiovascular Disease"

Key Terms

Watch for these terms and pay particular attention to what each one means, as you follow the textbook and video.

Oxygen starvation	**Thrombosis**
Pulmonary artery	**Embolism**
Aorta	**Heart attack/myocardial infarction**
Pacemaker	**Myocardial ischemia**
Arteries	**Angina pectoris**
Capillaries	**Coronary thrombosis**
Veins	**Coronary embolism**
Coronary arteries	**Cardiac arrest**
Carotid arteries and	**Collateral circulation**
Vertebral arteries	**Stroke**
Blood pressure	**Cerebral thrombosis**
Systolic pressure	**Cerebral embolism**
Diastolic pressure	**Cerebral hemorrhage**
Hypertension	**Transient ischemic attack (TIA)**
Atherosclerosis	**Arrythmia**
Plaque	**Ventricular fibrillation**
Thrombus	**Rheumatic fever**
Low density lipoproteins	**Congenital heart defects**
High density lipoproteins	**Congestive heart failure**
Ischemia	**Edema**

Text Focus Points

Before you read the textbook assignment, review the following points to help focus your thoughts. After you complete the assignment, write out your responses to reinforce what you have learned.

1. Describe the anatomy of the heart and circulatory system. Describe how blood flows through the heart and circulatory system.

2. What is blood pressure and how is it measured? Describe those who are at risk, the symptoms, and treatment of high blood pressure. Describe atherosclerosis, how it is caused, and the role of fats and cholesterol in its development. Describe disease conditions that can develop.

3. What is a heart attack? How does it happen? What are the symptoms? Explain the immediate actions that should be taken if someone experiences a heart attack, and the recovery process.

4. What is a stroke, and what are its symptoms? Briefly describe the recovery process.

5. Discuss the other major cardiovascular diseases: arrythmias, rheumatic heart disease, congenital heart defects, and congestive heart failure.

Experts Interviewed

In the video segment of this lesson, the following medical professionals share their expertise to help you understand the material presented.

Pamela S. Douglas, M.D., Director, Non-Invasive Cardiology, Beth Israel Hospital, Boston, Massachusetts, Associate Professor of Medicine, Harvard Medical School, Boston, Massachusetts

Richard Soltes, M.D., Internal Medicine, Dallas Diagnostic Association, Dallas, Texas

Video Focus Points

The following questions are designed to help you get the most from the video segment of this lesson. Review them before you watch the video. After viewing the video segment, write responses to reinforce what you have learned.

1. Explain the risk factors that increase one's chances of cardiovascular disease.

2. What changes in the cardiovascular system contribute to the actual heart attack?

Individual Health Plan

This portion of the lesson is designed to enable you to apply the information you have learned to your own life situation and improve the quality of your life. You should do any exercise assigned, complete the journal portion of the plan, then put this portion of the health plan into practice in your life.

Complete the self-assessment, "Estimate your RISKO Score for Heart Disease Risk," on pages 292-293 of the text. In your journal, describe some of your health practices that contribute to what you discovered about your risks. If you have controllable risks, develop a plan to lower these risks. Have your blood pressure checked several times over the semester and compare it with normal ranges. If you have doubts, consult your physician.

Enrichment Opportunity

This suggestion guides you if you want more information on this lesson, want to explore new ideas, or if your instructor requires it. If you are doing this section as a course requirement, consult with your instructor for specific guidelines or directions.

Contact your college Health Center, local American Heart Association, or American Red Cross and take a cardiopulmonary resuscitation (CPR) class.

Practice Test

After reading the assignment and watching the video, you should be able to answer the Practice Test questions. Tests also include essay questions that are similar to the Text Focus Points, the Video Focus Points, and the Objectives. When you have completed the Practice Test questions, turn to the Answer Key to score your answers..

1. Which parts of the heart work together as pumps?
   A. Ventricles and the atria
   B. Endocardium and the pericardium
   C. Aorta and the pulmonary artery
   D. Inferior and superior venae cavae

2. The blood makes a complete circuit of the circulatory system in approximately
   A. 10 - 15 seconds.
   B. 1 - 2 minutes.
   C. 3 - 5 minutes.
   D. 10 minutes.

3. The blood pressure recorded when the arteries are waiting for the next beat is called
   A. diastolic.
   B. systolic.
   C. pulse pressure.
   D. optimal.

4. Triglycerides and cholesterol are carried to the capillaries by
   A. low-density lipoproteins.
   B. triglycerides.
   C. high-density lipoproteins.
   D. all lipoproteins.

5. Myocardial ischemia is a condition in which a part of the heart is
   A. cut off from its blood supply.
   B. supplied too little blood and oxygen.
   C. overwhelmed with too much blood and oxygen.
   D. blocked by an embolus.

6. Stroke is LEAST likely to be described as
   A. sudden loss of brain function.
   B. resulting from interference of blood supply.
   C. cerebrovascular accident.
   D. untreatable illness of old age.

7. Which of the following statements is true of strokes?
   A. Strokes cannot be a direct cause of death.
   B. Strokes have the same symptoms as heart attacks.
   C. Strokes are always accompanied by acute pain.
   D. Strokes can vary widely in degree of severity.

8. Rheumatic fever often begins with
   A. influenza.
   B. strep throat.
   C. fungal infections.
   D. hepatitis.

9. Factors that place the individual at higher risk for cardiovascular disease include all the following EXCEPT
   A. smoking.
   B. high salt diet.
   C. sedentary lifestyle.
   D. low fat diet.

10. Cardiovascular changes that lead to disease include all the following EXCEPT
    A. narrowing vessels.
    B. increasing blood pressure.
    C. slowing heart rate.
    D. developing plaque.

11. Fatty deposits that can build up on the inner walls of blood vessels are called _____.

12. A swelling caused by fluid collecting in the tissues is called _____.

13. Lifestyle behaviors such as smoking and a high fat diet, which increase one's chances for cardiovascular disease, are termed _____.

14. When there is occlusion of the coronary arteries, the portion of the heart supplied by those arteries _____.

True or False

15. The blood is oxygenated (saturated with a fresh supply of oxygen) in the lungs.

16. After suffering a heart attack, the patient will never be able to resume an active life.

17. The causes of congenital heart defects are clearly understood.

18. A diet low in salt and high in fat can decrease the risk for cardiovascular disease.

19. Hypertension is quite different from high blood pressure and presents many symptoms as soon as it occurs.

20. Cardiovascular changes leading to a heart attack occur very suddenly.

Answer Key

These are the correct answers with reference to the Learning Objectives, and to the source of the information: the Textbook Focus Points, Levy, *et al. Life and Health,* and the Video Focus Points. Page numbers are also given for the Textbook Focus Points. KT indicates questions with Key Terms defined.

Question	Answer	Learning Objective	Textbook Focus Point (page no.)		Video Focus Point
1.	A	14.1	1 (p. 289)		
2.	A	14.1	1 (p. 289)		
3.	A	14.1	2 (p. 290)	KT	
4.	A	14.1	2 (p. 295)	KT	
5.	B	14.2	3 (p. 296)	KT	
6.	D	14.2	4 (p. 300)	KT	
7.	D	14.2	4 (p. 300)		
8.	B	14.2	5 (p. 304)	KT	
9.	D	14.1			1
10.	C	14.2			2
11.	plaque	14.1	2 (pp. 294-295)	KT	
12.	edema	14.2	5 (p. 305)	KT	
13.	risk factors	14.1			1
14.	dies	14.2			2
15.	T	14.1	1 (p. 289)		
16.	F	14.2	3 (p. 299)		
17.	F	14.2	5 (p. 304)		
18.	F	14.1			1
19.	F	14.1, 14.2			1
20.	F	14.2			2

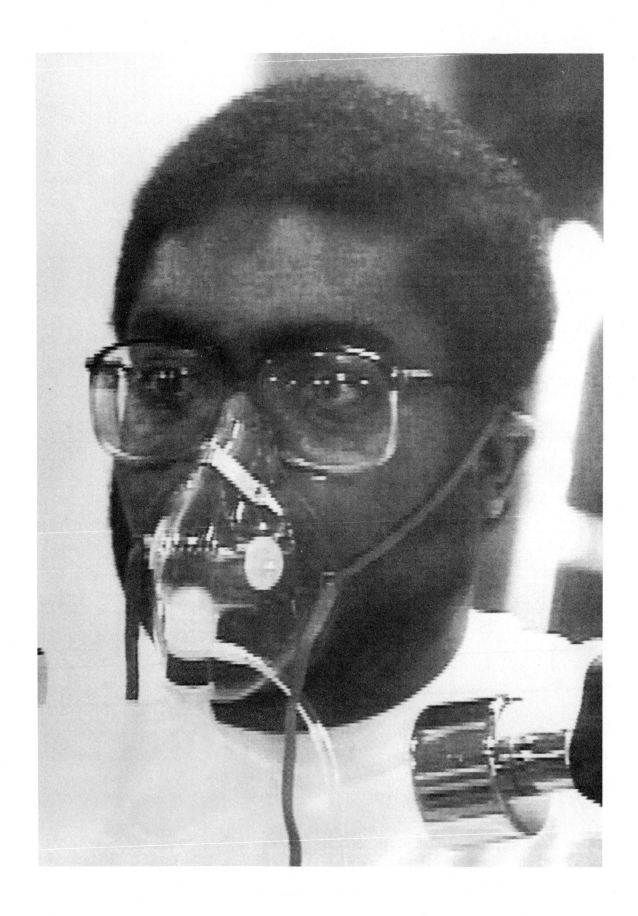

Lesson 15

Treatment and Prevention of Cardiovascular Disease

Perhaps the question we should ask ourselves is not 'Am I healthy?' but 'Am I as healthy as I know how to be?' I believe that for almost all persons the answer would be an unequivocal 'no.' Almost everyone knows how to implement a higher order of healthiness. And if a 'no' answer doesn't make us unmistakably uncomfortable, it is likely that we haven't squarely asked it. Answering 'no' means we have hidden from ourselves. We have shunned an inner wisdom.

Larry Dossey, M.D., *Beyond Illness*

Overview

While modern medicine has brought much hope for victims of cardiovascular disease, the most important treatment is actual prevention of the problem. Nowhere are our lifestyle decisions more important than in this group of diseases. While some of our risk factors are uncontrollable, most of those things that put us at higher risk for cardiovascular diseases can be controlled. Of even more concern is the way in which risk factors tend to multiply and reinforce each other. Somehow, if we have one bad lifestyle habit, we tend to have several which impact each other. If we are overweight, we tend not to exercise. If we smoke, we smoke even more when we are under stress. The good news is that good lifestyle habits tend to reinforce each other as well. When we exercise and eat in a healthy way, we lose weight and frequently handle stress more effectively.

The sooner we make decisions to improve our health, the sooner we lower our risks for cardiovascular and other diseases. Bad habits can be difficult to break, but if we do not become discouraged, we will reap the benefits of our work. We don't even have to do all things at once. We can work on our risks one by one. The important thing is that we begin. We will feel better, be healthier, and will have less risk of developing cardiovascular problems.

Learning Objectives

Goal: You should be able to identify and discuss methods of treatment of cardiovascular diseases and lifestyle behaviors that lower the risk of cardiovascular disease.

Objectives: Upon completion of this lesson, you should be able to:

1. Identify and discuss the tests and treatments for cardiovascular disease which are used the most frequently.

2. Discuss the uncontrollable and controllable risk factors for cardiovascular disease, the danger of multiple risk factors, and how the controllable risk factors can be reduced.

Study Assignments

Pay careful attention to the following assignments. The chapter number may not be the same as the lesson number.

Textbook: Chapter 11, "Cardiovascular Health and Disease", pp. 301-303, 305-311

Video: "Treatment and Prevention of Cardiovascular Disease"

Key Terms

Watch for these terms and pay particular attention to what each one means, as you follow the textbook and video.

Angioplasty
Bypass surgery

Text Focus Points

Before you read the textbook assignment, review the following points to help focus your thoughts. After you complete the assignment, write out your responses to reinforce what you have learned.

1. Identify and describe tests for the early diagnosis of cardiovascular disease.

2. Discuss several of the most common treatments for cardiovascular disease.

3. What are the uncontrollable and controllable risk factors for cardiovascular disease and how can controllable risk factors be reduced? What effects does tobacco smoking have on the heart and circulatory system? What is the link between obesity and coronary heart disease?

4. Explain why the presence of multiple risk factors poses a greater danger with cardiovascular disease.

Expert Interviewed

In the video segment of this lesson, the following medical professional shares his expertise to help you understand the material presented.

Reginald L. Washington, M.D., Vice President, Rocky Mountain Pediatric Cardiology, P.C., Denver, Colorado

Video Focus Points

The following questions are designed to help you get the most from the video segment of this lesson. Review them before you watch the video. After viewing the video segment, write responses to reinforce what you have learned.

1. Why is having the knowledge of cardiopulmonary resuscitation (CPR) so important to the individual?

2. Discuss the various treatments for cardiovascular disease: medication, angioplasty, bypass surgery, and transplant.

3. What are some of the emotional and physical aspects involved in recovery from a heart attack?

4. What lifestyle choices and behaviors are important in lowering the individual's risk for cardiovascular disease? How are these important?

Individual Health Plan

This portion of the lesson is designed to enable you to apply the information you have learned to your own life situation and improve the quality of your life. You should do any exercise assigned, complete the journal portion of the plan, then put this portion of the health plan into practice in your life.

After assessing your risk factors for cardiovascular disease, in your journal develop a plan for lowering these risks using information you have gained in this lesson. Take action on your plan today.

Enrichment Opportunity

This suggestion guides you if you want more information on this lesson, want to explore new ideas, or if your instructor requires it. If you are doing this section as a course requirement, consult with your instructor for specific guidelines or directions.

Design a cardiovascular risk reduction for your own family based on your individual and family risks.

Practice Test

After reading the assignment and watching the video, you should be able to answer the Practice Test questions. Tests also include essay questions that are similar to the Text Focus Points, the Video Focus Points, and the Objectives. When you have completed the Practice Test questions, turn to the Answer Key to score your answers.

---

1. In by-pass surgery,
   A. sections of the heart are transplanted.
   B. part of a coronary artery is replaced.
   C. diameter of the coronary artery is increased.
   D. valves in the heart are replaced.

2. Which of the following factors increases one's risks of developing cardiovascular disease?
   A. Smoking
   B. Low-cholesterol diet
   C. Reduced fat diet
   D. Aerobic exercise

3. Risk of heart attack is erroneously assumed to be lower for
   A. older than for younger people.
   B. women than for men.
   C. whites than for African-Americans or Asians.
   D. sedentary individuals rather than individuals who exercise regularly.

4. Effects of tobacco smoking do NOT include
   A. speeding heart rate.
   B. raising blood pressure.
   C. constricting blood vessels.
   D. slowing the heart rate.

5. When present in combination, cardiovascular risk factors interact
   A. to reduce overall risk.
   B. synergistically to multiply the risk.
   C. as they would if present one at a time.
   D. not at all.

6. Cardiopulmonary resuscitation (CPR) should be learned by
   A. health care professionals.
   B. food service workers.
   C. everyone.
   D. police and fire officers.

7. When the heart is damaged beyond repair, the patient may have to consider
   A. open heart repair.
   B. heart transplant.
   C. angioplasty.
   D. bypass surgery.

8. After a heart attack, the individual frequently has all the following EXCEPT
   A. few emotional concerns.
   B. changed dietary habits.
   C. significant physical rehabilitation.
   D. lifestyle adjustments.

9. Hypertension is the same thing as
   A. hyperactivity.
   B. angioplasty.
   C. atherosclerosis.
   D. high blood pressure.

10. Tests that chart the electrical activity of the heart to reveal cardiovascular abnormalities are called _____.

11. When a balloon-type apparatus is threaded through the blood vessels to remove a blockage, the procedure is known as _____.

12. The procedure in which the heart is removed and replaced by one from another person is called _____.

True or False
13. Most of the tests for cardiovascular disease are painless and can be done on an outpatient basis.

14. There is no relationship between family history of cardiovascular disease and risk of heart attack.

15. Though hypertension is a serious problem, no relationship exists between high blood pressure and stroke or heart attack.

16. If an individual has several risk factors for cardiovascular disease, correcting them all at once is easiest.

Lesson 16

Cancer

I'm living today with as much empowerment as I can and trying to help others. . . . I'm taking today a day at a time and I feel very good about that, so how much future does anybody have, mine's as good as yours.

Beatrice Quintero, Cancer Survivor

Overview

When people think of cancer, they frequently experience fear and think of cancer as a death sentence. This is just not true, though too many people are still dying of cancer. We need to understand that most cancers are treatable, and many are curable. Even more important to us, many cancers are preventable. Practicing a lifestyle that minimizes our risk factors for cancer can decrease our chance of dying of cancer dramatically. These lifestyle behaviors that put us at risk for cancer are similar to the ones that place us at risk for other health problems: tobacco, alcohol, poor dietary habits, the use of certain drugs, and exposure to certain carcinogenic substances.

Of equal importance to us is the knowledge of the seven warning signs of cancer and the key role that early detection plays in the treatment of cancer. One of the real tragedies of cancer is that people often delay getting treatment. There are several reasons for this delay: fear, not recognizing the early warning signs, not practicing self-examination, etc. But whatever the reason, delay in detection and treatment decreases our chances for successful treatment and survival of cancer. If we are to maximize our chances of preventing cancer, as well as surviving it should we get it, we must first practice a healthy lifestyle that lowers our risk for the disease. We must know the seven warning signs and practice self-examination. Then if we experience symptoms that indicate any possibility of cancer, we must seek diagnosis and treatment from a qualified physician immediately! If we do these things we increase our chance for a healthy, cancer-free life dramatically!

Learning Objectives

Goal: You should be able to describe cancer, its various types, metastatic growth, the importance of early detection, treatment of cancer, and lifestyle behaviors that decrease the risk of cancer.

Objectives: Upon completion of this lesson, you should be able to:

1. Explain the significance of cancer as a leading cause of death, reasons that deaths from cancer are increasing, and the emotional and social effects of cancer.

2. Discuss what cancer is, the various types of cancer, the process of metastatic growth, the risk factors and methods for reducing the risk for cancer.

3. Discuss the importance of early detection in cancer treatment, the seven warning signs of cancer, self-examination procedures, and ways in which people can cope with cancer.

4. Describe the importance of staging in determining the treatment of cancer, the most common methods of treating cancer, and some of the newer methods being developed to treat cancer.

Study Assignments

Textbook: Chapter 12, "Cancer: Some Cause for Hope," pp. 312-334

Video: "Cancer"

Key Terms

Watch for these terms and pay particular attention to what each one means, as you follow the textbook and video.

Cancer or malignant neoplasm	**Epithelium**
Mitosis	**Sarcomas**
Tumor	**Adenocarcinomas**
Neoplasm	**Lymphomas**
Benign tumor	**Leukemias**
Malignant tumor	**Melanoma**
Metastases	**Anaplastic**
Metastatic growth	**Carcinogenic**
Carcinoma	

Text Focus Points

Before you read the textbook assignment, review the following points to help focus your thoughts. After you complete the assignment, write out your responses to reinforce what you have learned.

1. What is the significance of cancer as a leading cause of death in the United States today and why has the death rate increased? Is there any cause for hope?

2. Explain what cancer is, the process of metastatic growth, and the various types of cancer.

3. Discuss the emotional and social effects of cancer on people.

4. What are the most important risk factors for cancer and how can people reduce their risk for cancer?

5. Explain the importance of early detection in cancer treatment and describe the procedures for self-examination. Include the seven warning signs of cancer.

6. Explain the goals of staging in assessing treatment for cancer and discuss the primary treatments used for treating cancer. Include some of the new developments in diagnosis and treatment and the dangers of quackery.

7. Can a person be cured of cancer? Discuss some of the ways people attempt to cope with cancer and explain how cancer patients can be helped to cope with the disease.

Experts Interviewed

In the video segment of this lesson, the following medical and health professionals share their expertise to help you understand the material presented.

James W. Bowen, Ph.D., Vice President for Academic Affairs, Professor of Virology, The University of Texas M.D. Anderson Cancer Center, Houston, Texas

Judy A. Gerner, Director, Anderson Network, The University of Texas M.D. Anderson Cancer Center, Houston, Texas

Bernard Levin, M.D., Vice President for Cancer Prevention (ad interim), Chairman, Department of Gastrointestinal Medical Oncology and Digestive Diseases, The University of Texas M.D. Anderson Cancer Center, Houston, Texas

S. Eva Singletary, M.D., Associate Professor of Surgical Oncology, The University of Texas M.D. Anderson Cancer Center, Houston, Texas

Video Focus Points

The following questions are designed to help you get the most from the video segment of this lesson. Review them before you watch the video. After viewing the video segment, write responses to reinforce what you have learned.

1. Explain what cancer is, the major types of cancer, and how cancer spreads.

2. Explain the circumstances under which the three most common types of cancer treatment are used.

3. Describe three kinds of emotional issues cancer patients and their families must face relative to each patient's attitude toward treatment.

4. Discuss eight lifestyle behaviors that will decrease the individual's risk of cancer.

Individual Health Plan

This portion of the lesson is designed to enable you to apply the information you have learned in your own life situation and improve the quality of your life. You should do any exercise assigned, complete the journal portion of the plan, then put this portion of the health plan into practice in your life.

In your journal, list your own lifestyle behaviors that increase or decrease your risk for cancer. On the basis of what you have learned in this unit, develop and write a plan for lowering your own risk of dying of cancer. Once you have developed this plan, put it into effect.

Enrichment Opportunity

These suggestions guide you if you want more information on this lesson, want to explore new ideas, or if your instructor requires it. If you are doing this section as a course requirement, consult with your instructor for specific guidelines or directions.

Visit the local chapter of the American Cancer Society to find out what educational material and community services it provides. Consider volunteering in a program.

Practice Test

After reading the assignment and watching the video, you should be able to answer the Practice Test questions. Tests also include essay questions that are similar to the Text Focus Points, the Video Focus Points, and the Objectives. When you have completed the Practice Test questions, turn to the Answer Key to score your answers.

1. Since 1900, the death rate from cancer has
   A. greatly increased.
   B. greatly decreased.
   C. remained the same.
   D. fluctuated.

2. Cancer cells are NOT characterized by
   A. inability to function as intended.
   B. rapid growth.
   C. increased rate of reproduction.
   D viral infection.

3. Which of the following is NOT a common emotional response to a diagnosis of cancer?
   A. Anorexia nervosa
   B. Anxiety
   C. Depression
   D. Anger

4. At highest risk for developing skin cancer are individuals with
   A. leukemia.
   B. sarcoma.
   C. dark complexions.
   D. fair complexions.

5. Today, the greatest hope for cancer patients lies in
   A. discovery of antibodies.
   B. radiation therapy.
   C. early detection.
   D. chemotherapy.

6. The procedure by which a physician evaluates the type of treatment best suited for a patient at a given time is called
   A. chemotherapy.
   B. psychotherapy.
   C. staging.
   D. psychosurgery.

7. Which of the following phrases does NOT describe cancer?
   A. Group of diseases
   B. Generally untreatable
   C. Capable of metastatic growth
   D. Problem of regulation and differentiation of cells

8. Most cancers are treated using
   A. surgery.
   B. radiation.
   C. chemotherapy.
   D. combinations of treatments.

9. Which of the following lifestyle behaviors will NOT decrease the risk of cancer?
   A. Not smoking
   B. Abstaining from alcohol
   C. Getting a good suntan
   D. Eating a high fiber diet

10. Cancers of blood-forming cells are known as _____.

11. Foods that are high in fiber seem to have a protective effect against cancer of the _____.

12. The use of chemicals to treat cancer is called _____.

13. Cancers that arise in the blood forming tissues are leukemias and _____.

14. A test which contributes to lowering the risk of dying from breast cancer is the _____.

True or False
15. Today's technology and medical techniques permit earlier, more accurate diagnosis of cancer than was possible in the past.

16. For some cancer patients, the fear of dying is probably unrealistic.

17. Most tumors are detected first by physicians examining the patient.

18. Once a person survives cancer for five years, they are no longer at risk.

19. Localized tumors are usually treated with chemotherapy.

20. When the diagnosis of cancer is made, most people respond with shock, denial, or even anger.

Answer Key

These are the correct answers with reference to the Learning Objectives, and to the source of the information: the Textbook Focus Points, Levy, *et al. Life and Health,* and the Video Focus Points. Page numbers are also given for the Textbook Focus Points. KT indicates questions with Key Terms defined.

Question	Answer	Learning Objective	Textbook Focus Point (page no.)	Video Focus Point
1.	A	16.1	1 (p. 313)	
2.	D	16.2	2 (pp. 314-315) .... KT	
3.	A	16.1	3 (pp. 317-318)	
4.	D	16.2	4 (p. 318)	
5.	C	16.3	5 (p. 322)	
6.	C	16.4	6 (p. 326)	
7.	B	16.2		1
8.	D	16.4		2
9.	C	16.2		4
10.	leukemias	16.2	2 (p. 316) .... KT	
11.	colon	16.2	4 (p. 321)	
12.	chemotherapy	16.4	6 (p. 328)	
13.	lymphomas	16.2		1
14.	mammogram	16.2		4
15.	T	16.1	1 (p. 313)	
16.	T	16.1	3 (p. 317)	
17.	F	16.3	5 (p. 323)	
18.	F	16.3	7 (p. 331)	
19.	F	16.4		2
20.	T	16.1		3

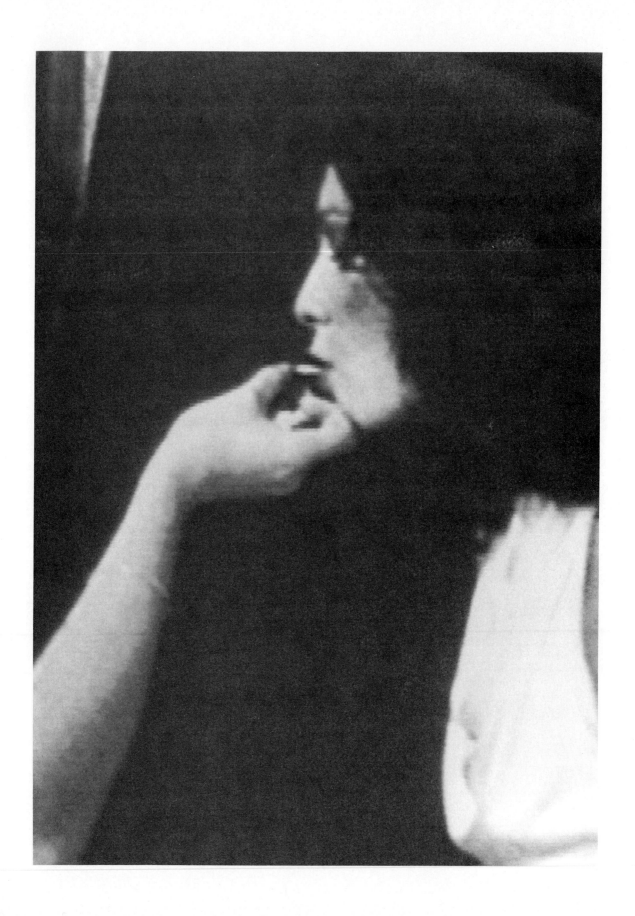

Lesson 17

Drugs

The mental and spiritual qualities of man will never be dignified through debasing the physical and vice versa. This understanding is crucial to the maturation of a holistic theory of health . . . .

Larry Dossey, M.D., *Beyond Illness*

Overview

At the same time that we are so concerned with drug abuse, we must look at the environment in which this abuse is taking place. We have to face the fact that we are a drug-oriented society. All we have to do is turn on our television or open a magazine to realize that "there is a pill for everything." While many drugs save lives and are absolutely necessary to our health and well-being, some of these and many others are overused, misused, abused and present major health problems.

Many of the reasons that cause people to misuse and abuse drugs, including alcohol, relate to two concepts. One is the relief of pain whether it be physical, emotional, or social. The other is an attempt to make life different, to be accepted, to fit in, to be happy, etc. If we consider this, we will see that there are always more positive means to achieve these objectives. This is what making healthy lifestyle decisions is all about. Coping with the ups and downs of life certainly is not always easy, but while drug use may seem a simple solution for the present, it creates havoc in the longer term. The negative health effects on the individual, his or her family, and even future generations is just not worth the momentary high.

Drug misuse and abuse crosses all socio-economic, ethnic, gender, and age lines. There is not a typical drug abuser. No one is "immune" to the risk. If you or someone you care about is having a problem, get help. Now is the time for each of us to take the responsibility for making decisions for health. In addition to preventing or solving problems for ourselves, we can help solve a greater community problem because as the demand for drugs decreases, so does the illegal drug trade and its societal problems.

Learning Objectives

Goal: You should be able to discuss the various aspects of drug use, the agent-host-environment model in relationship to drug use, risks of drug abuse, and positive alternatives to drug use.

Objectives: Upon completion of this lesson, you should be able to:

1. Define drugs and describe some of the uses for prescription drugs and how drugs affect the body.

2. Discuss drug use including the relationship of the agent-host-environment model, reasons for drug use, tolerance, dependence, addiction, and the significance of the various levels of drug use.

3. Explain how drugs affect the body, the ways drugs are administered, the time-response relationship, the dose-response relationship, and possible problems with drug interactions.

4. Explain the effects and potential risks of each group of major psychoactive drugs and other drugs of abuse.

5. Discuss the way in which society deals with drug use and abuse, ways of dealing with the need for drugs, and the types of treatment programs that exist.

Study Assignments

Pay careful attention to the following assignments. The chapter number may not be the same as the lesson number.

Textbook: Chapter 13, "Drug Use and Abuse," pp. 336-369

Video: "Drugs"

Key Terms

Watch for these terms and pay particular attention to what each one means, as you follow the textbook and video.

Drug	Therapeutic index
Psychoactive drug	Synergism
Nonpsychoactive	Sedatives/hypnotics
Tolerance	Stimulants
Dependence	Amphetamines
Withdrawal syndrome	Cocaine
Addiction	Marijuana
Receptor theory	Inhalants
Receptor sites	Amyl nitrite
Side effects	Butyl nitrite
Teratogenic	Opiate narcotics
Allergy	Opiates
Anaphylactic shock	Opium
Cross-sensitivity	Morphine
Route of administration	Heroin
Subcutaneous	"Tango and cash"
Intramuscular	Psychedelics/hallucinogens
Intravenous	Detoxification
Biotransform	Methadone
Metabolites	

Text Focus Points

Before you read the textbook assignment, review the following points to help focus your thoughts. After you complete the assignment, write out your responses to reinforce what you have learned.

1. What are drugs and what is the difference between psychoactive and nonpsychoactive drugs? What are some of the uses for prescription drugs?

2. Distinguish between tolerance, dependence, and addiction.

3. How do people become dependent on drugs? Include a discussion of the significance of the various levels of drug use.

4. Explain the agent-host-environment model as it pertains to drug use. Include discussion of trends in drug use.

5. Describe how drugs interact with body cells and how drugs affect the body.

6. Identify and describe the primary ways in which drugs are administered. What are the disadvantages of inhalation?

7. Explain the time-response relationship and the dose-response relationship. Distinguish between effective and lethal doses.

8. Describe the types of drug interactions. What can happen if alcohol is combined with sedatives?

9. List the major psychoactive drugs and explain some of their effects and potential risks.

10. What are some ways of dealing with the need for drugs and what types of treatment programs exist?

Experts Interviewed

In the video segment of this lesson, the following medical and health professionals share their expertise to help you understand the material presented.

Cheryé C. Callegan, M.D., Chief, Substance Abuse Services, Timberlawn Psychiatric Hospital, Dallas, Texas

J. Pat Evans, M.D., Medical Director, Tom Landry Sports Medicine and Research Center, Dallas, Texas

Thomas R. Kosten, M.D., Associate Professor of Psychiatry, Yale University School of Medicine, New Haven, Connecticut

Video Focus Points

The following questions are designed to help you get the most from the video segment of this lesson. Review them before you watch the video. After viewing the video segment, write responses to reinforce what you have learned.

1. Describe the risks of and alternatives to anabolic steroid use.

2. Discuss the problems of drug abuse in society today. What are some of the decisions that have to be made if the problems of drug abuse are to be solved?

3. What are the risks of and problems associated with the interaction of alcohol with other drugs and combinations of drugs?

Individual Health Plan

This portion of the lesson is designed to enable you to apply the information you have learned to your own life situation and improve the quality of your life. You should do any exercise assigned, complete the journal portion of the plan, then put this portion of the health plan into practice in your life.

> In your journal, examine the role that drugs play in your life. Consider the positive uses (antibiotics, etc.) as well as possible negatives. Include caffeine and any other "every day" substance that you might not think of as a drug. Are there changes you should make to be healthier? What decisions will you need to make? What are some positive alternatives? If you feel that you are having a problem, consult your physician, your college health center or your local Council on Alcoholism and Drug Abuse.

Enrichment Opportunity

This suggestion guides you if you want more information on this lesson, want to explore new ideas, or if your instructor requires it. If you are doing this section as a course requirement, consult with your instructor for specific guidelines or directions.

> Visit several drug treatment centers in your city and find out about their programs. Compare and contrast their approaches, costs, etc.

Practice Test

After reading the assignment and watching the video, you should be able to answer the Practice Test questions. Tests also include essay questions that are similar to the Text Focus Points, the Video Focus Points, and the Objectives. When you have completed the Practice Test questions, turn to the Answer Key to score your answers.

1. Marijuana and cocaine are examples of
   A. psychoactive drugs.
   B. nonpsychoactive drugs.
   C. opiates.
   D. barbiturates.

2. A compulsive pattern of drug use, with the person dependent on the drug both physically and psychologically, is termed
   A. dependence.
   B. tolerance.
   C. addiction.
   D. habituation.

3. When individuals use drugs to experience effects they consider beneficial in certain circumstances, they are engaging in use of drugs referred to as
   A. intensified.
   B. compulsive.
   C. situational.
   D. recreational.

4. The major cause of side effects of drugs is the fact that some
   A. users do not follow directions.
   B. prescribing physicians use poor judgment.
   C. drugs are less selective about attaching to receptor sites.
   D. food substances interact with certain drugs.

5. Which of the following statements is true of drug doses?
   A. The lethal dose of a drug is five times its effective dose.
   B. Many individuals do not respond to the effective dose.
   C. Anyone who takes the lethal dose of a drug will die.
   D. Some drugs have no lethal dose.

6. When alcohol is combined with barbiturates, the effects of each drug are
   A. blocked out.
   B. diminished.
   C. increased.
   D. transformed.

7. Drugs that activate the sympathetic division of the autonomic nervous system, causing restlessness, talkativeness, and inability to sleep, are known as
   A. psychedelics.
   B. phencyclidines.
   C. stimulants.
   D. volatile solvents.

8. Risks of anabolic steroids do NOT include
   A. cancer of the liver.
   B. heart problems.
   C. personality disorders.
   D. tuberculosis.

9. Categories for describing usage of drugs would NOT include
   A. biological.
   B. medical.
   C. social/psychological.
   D. political.

10. The interaction of sedative/tranquilizer drugs and alcohol causes
    A. each drug to be less effective.
    B. significant potentiation/synergistic effects.
    C. very predictable effects.
    D. no problem that either drug would not cause by itself.

11. The type of shock resulting from an allergic reaction to a drug in which blood pressure drops to a dangerous level is known as _____.

12. A drug injection directly into a vein is termed _____.

13. The desire for heroin can be removed through the use of the synthetic drug known as _____.

14. The genetic predisposition of an individual to abuse drugs is a
_____.

True or False

15. Psychoactive drugs have much more potential for abuse than do other drugs.

16. Emotional problems are environmental factors in the agent-host environment model of drug dependence.

17. Even though cola drinks contain caffeine, no real concern about consumption by children is needed.

18. Most anabolic steroid use occurs among college and professional athletes.

19. The incidence of drug abuse is lower among individuals who come from dysfunctional families.

20. Most times, the effects of the interaction of alcohol and other depressant drugs is just slightly greater than the effect of either drug alone.

Answer Key

These are the correct answers with reference to the Learning Objectives, and to the source of the information: the Textbook Focus Points, Levy, *et al. Life and Health,* and the Video Focus Points. Page numbers are also given for the Textbook Focus Points. KT indicates questions with Key Terms defined.

Question	Answer	Learning Objective	Textbook Focus Point (page no.)		Video Focus Point
1.	A	17.1	1 (p. 338)		
2.	C	17.2	2 (p. 340)	KT	
3.	C	17.2	3 (p. 341)		
4.	C	17.1, 17.3	5 (p. 345)	KT	
5.	B	17.3	7 (p. 348)		
6.	C	17.3	8 (pp. 349-350)		
7.	C	17.4	9 (p. 356)	KT	
8.	D	17.5			1
9.	D	17.5			2
10.	B	17.3			3
11.	anaphylactic	17.1, 17.3	5 (p. 346)	KT	
12.	intravenous	17.3	6 (p. 347)	KT	
13.	methadone	17.5	10 (p. 366)	KT	
14.	biological factor	17.5			2
15.	T	17.1	1 (p. 338)		
16.	F	17.2	4 (p. 342)		
17.	F	17.4	9 (p. 357)		
18.	F	17.5			1
19.	F	17.5			2
20.	F	17.3			3

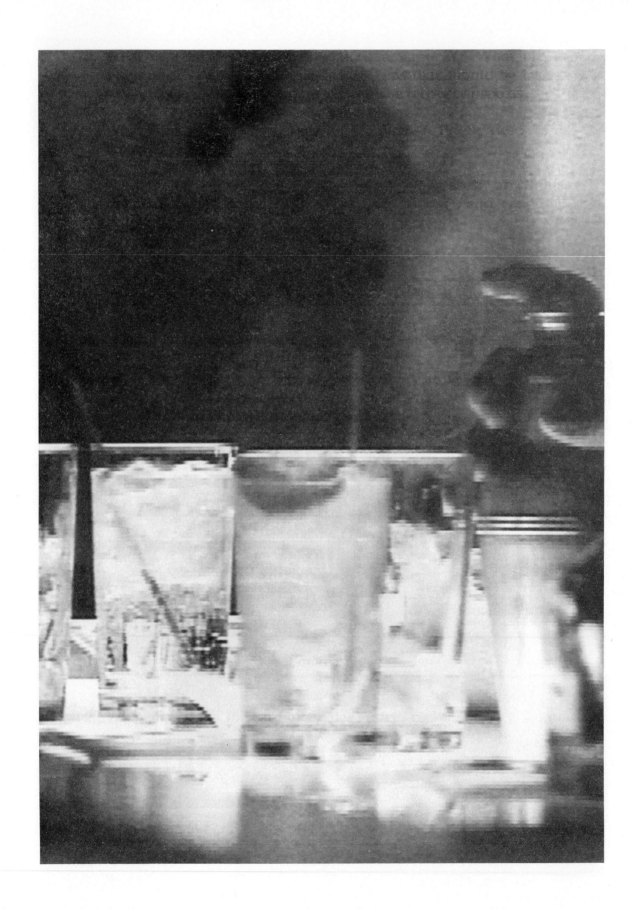

Lesson 18

Alcohol

In American society, one of the biggest factors that contributes to people drinking is that alcohol is not seen as a drug. It's in some ways seen as a rite of passage.

Robin LaDue, Ph.D.

Overview

Alcohol has a strange history. On one hand it is accepted and even expected at many celebrations, on the other, it is the most abused of all drugs and causes enormous health problems. The obvious question is, "Why?" Why do some people use alcohol all their lives without experiencing any difficulties while others develop problems of great magnitude? The answers are varied and complex. What we do know is that excessive use of alcohol, even minimal amounts (as in the case of the pregnant woman) can cause significant damage to most body systems. Alcohol also plays an important role in violence of all kinds, from motor vehicle accidents to murder.

To make decisions about our own lifestyle in relationship to alcohol, it is important for us to understand the effects of alcohol on the body. Alcohol acts as an anesthetic, a sedative, and a depressant. This means that even small amounts are risky if we are doing anything that requires us to be alert. Small amounts of alcohol can also damage the developing fetus, so pregnant women are encouraged to abstain from alcohol use. A decision not to use alcohol certainly lowers our risk for problems, but it is also possible to use alcohol responsibly if we choose to. The important thing is that if we use alcohol, we use it responsibly so as not to cause harm to ourselves or others.

It has been said that you have an alcohol problem if your use of alcohol causes problems to you, your loved ones, your job, or any aspect of your life. This is a good measure if you think you or someone you care about seems to be developing alcohol problems. If you suspect alcohol problems may exist, there are many places to get help. Alcoholics Anonymous is the best known, but most cities have a variety of options for seeking help.

If you understand the effects and potential risks of alcohol use, you can make wise lifestyle decisions, whether you choose to abstain from alcohol or use alcohol in a responsible way.

Learning Objectives

Goal: You should be able to explain the significance of alcohol use in this country, the factors that influence alcohol use, the health and behavior consequences of alcohol abuse, and the responsible use of alcohol.

Objectives: Upon completion of this lesson, you should be able to:

1. Explain the history and significance of drug use in this country, the factors that influence alcohol use, and the relationship of alcohol use and destructive behavior.

2. Describe the way alcohol affects the body, the health consequences of chronic alcohol use, the steps in the development of alcoholism, signs of potential alcoholism, and treatment of alcoholism.

3. Discuss the responsible use of alcohol and possible alternatives to alcohol use.

Study Assignments

Pay careful attention to the following assignments. The chapter number may not be the same as the lesson number.

Textbook: Chapter, 14, "Alcohol," pp. 370-387

Video: "Alcohol"

Key Terms

Watch for these terms and pay particular attention to what each one means, as you follow the textbook and video.

Ethyl alcohol	**Blackout**
Blood alcohol level (BAL)	**Pancreatitis**
Hangover	**Cirrhosis of the liver**
Tolerance	**Alcoholic hepatitis**
Alcoholism	**Detoxification**

Text Focus Points

Before you read the textbook assignment, review the following points to help focus your thoughts. After you complete the assignment, write out your responses to reinforce what you have learned.

1. Discuss the significance and history of alcohol use in this country.

2. Describe how alcohol travels through the body. Explain how the amount of food eaten and body size influence the effects of alcohol. Describe the effects of alcohol on the central nervous system. Why is alcohol seen as a stimulant?

3. Explain the factors that influence alcohol use and the relationship between alcohol abuse and different types of destructive behavior.

4. Define alcoholism. Describe the progressive steps in the development of alcoholism and identify signs and causes of potential alcoholism. What are the trends of alcoholism among men and women?

5. What are some of the major health consequences of chronic, excessive alcohol use. Discuss each.

6. Discuss the ways people can use alcohol responsibly.

---

7. Explain the most commonly used methods of treating alcoholism, including Alcoholics Anonymous.

8. Describe possible alternatives to alcohol use.

Expert Interviewed

In the video segment of this lesson, the following health professional shares her expertise to help you understand the material presented.

Robin A. LaDue, Ph.D., Clinical Psychologist, Fetal Alcohol and Drug Unit, University of Washington Medical School, Seattle, Washington

Video Focus Points

The following questions are designed to help you get the most from the video segment of this lesson. Review them before you watch the video. After viewing the video segment, write responses to reinforce what you have learned.

1. Describe how social and psychological factors influence alcohol use and can place the individual consuming alcohol at risk.

2. Describe the progression toward alcoholism and some of the signs of alcoholism.

3. How is alcohol related to accidents and other violence?

4. What are some important considerations in the responsible use of alcohol?

Individual Health Plan

This portion of the lesson is designed to enable you to apply the information you have learned in your own life situation and improve the quality of your life. You should do any exercise assigned, complete the journal portion of the plan, then put this portion of the health plan into practice in your life.

After comparing your own alcohol use with the levels in "Comfort Level" in your text, page 383, record your findings in your journal. Are there things that surprise you? Concern you? What did you learn about your patterns of alcohol use? If you found that there are times that you use alcohol irresponsibly, what will it take to change this pattern? Consider making some responsible decisions. If you discovered things that concerned you, discuss these with your college counseling or health center staff, your physician, or some other health professional.

Note: If you do not use alcohol, discuss the reasons that led you to make the decision to abstain from alcohol use.

Enrichment Opportunities

These suggestions guide you if you want more information on this lesson, want to explore new ideas, or if your instructor requires it. If you are doing this section as a course requirement, consult with your instructor for specific guidelines or directions.

1. Visit an open AA meeting and find out how the concept of a 12-step program works.

2. Contact several alcohol treatment programs and find how they treat alcohol abuse.

3. Interview a recovering alcoholic and find out how their life has progressed before, during, and since their alcohol abuse.

Practice Test

After reading the assignment and watching the video, you should be able to answer the Practice Test questions. Tests also include essay questions that are similar to the Text Focus Points, the Video Focus Points, and the Objectives. When you have completed the Practice Test questions, turn to the Answer Key to score your answers.

1. After the passage of the Prohibition amendment, the demand for alcohol
   A. increased.
   B. remained high.
   C. decreased.
   D. dropped to zero.

2. Most individuals will become drunk more quickly if they drink
   A. when relaxed.
   B. at night.
   C. after eating a full meal.
   D. on an empty stomach.

3. Which of the following statements is true of alcohol?
   A. Individuals cannot develop a tolerance to alcohol.
   B. Some individuals can develop a physical dependence on alcohol.
   C. Individuals cannot develop a psychic dependence on alcohol.
   D. Some individuals are immune to the effects of alcohol.

4. An individual who drinks to intoxication and gets drunk without intending to is
   A. an occasional drinker.
   B. a light drinker.
   C. a social drinker.
   D. a problem drinker.

5. Which of the following is a gastrointestinal disorder sometimes related to alcohol use?
   A. Impotence
   B. Cirrhosis
   C. Ulcer
   D. Malnutrition

6. Alcoholics Anonymous members begin their treatment by admitting that they
   A. enjoy alcohol.
   B. lost control over alcohol.
   C. profess deep religious beliefs.
   D. feel malnourished.

7. Reasons that people begin drinking do NOT include
   A. peer pressure.
   B. rite of passage.
   C. taste of alcohol.
   D. advertising.

8. A major sign that alcohol is becoming a problem is
   A. functioning level at work.
   B. drinking on the weekend.
   C. consuming hard liquor.
   D. acknowledging the problem within the family.

9. After it is consumed, alcohol travels to the stomach and to the
   _____.

10. The individual who drinks on special occasions to be sociable, the first stage in the alcohol continuum, is referred to as the _____ drinker.

11. The disease in which the liver becomes swollen and inflamed is known as alcoholic _____.

12. Treatment of alcoholism generally concentrates first on the aspects of the illness which are _____.

13. The various stages of progression to alcoholism is called the alcoholic _____.

True or False

14. Blood alcohol level is the amount of alcohol that is in the blood at one time.

15. Alcohol plays a key role in motor vehicle accidents.

16. Although the incidence of alcoholism is higher in men than in women, the incidence in women is rising.

17. People rarely begin to drink before young adulthood.

18. The tendency to progress toward alcoholism is limited to a narrow segment of the population.

19. Alcohol is involved in many motor vehicle accidents, but plays a lesser role in other violence.

20. Responsible use of alcohol can mean that the person abstains from alcohol completely.

Answer Key

These are the correct answers with reference to the Learning Objectives, and to the source of the information: the Textbook Focus Points, Levy, *et al. Life and Health,* and the Video Focus Points. Page numbers are also given for the Textbook Focus Points. KT indicates questions with Key Terms defined.

Question	Answer	Learning Objective	Textbook Focus Point (page no.)	Video Focus Point
1.	B	18.1	1 (p. 371)	
2.	D	18.2	2 (pp. 372-373)	
3.	B	18.1	3 (p. 374)	
4.	D	18.2	4 (p. 377)	
5.	C	18.2	5 (p. 379)	
6.	B	18.2	7 (p. 385)	
7.	C	18.1		1
8.	D	18.2		2
9.	small intestine	18.2	2 (p. 372)	
10.	occasional	18.2	4 (p. 377)	
11.	hepatitis	18.2	5 (p. 381)	KT
12.	physical	18.2	7 (p. 384)	
13.	continuum	18.2		2
14.	T	18.2	2 (p. 373)	KT
15.	T	18.1	3 (p. 375)	
16.	T	18.2	4 (p. 379)	
17.	F	18.1		1
18.	F	18.2		2
19.	F	18.1		3
20.	T	18.3		4

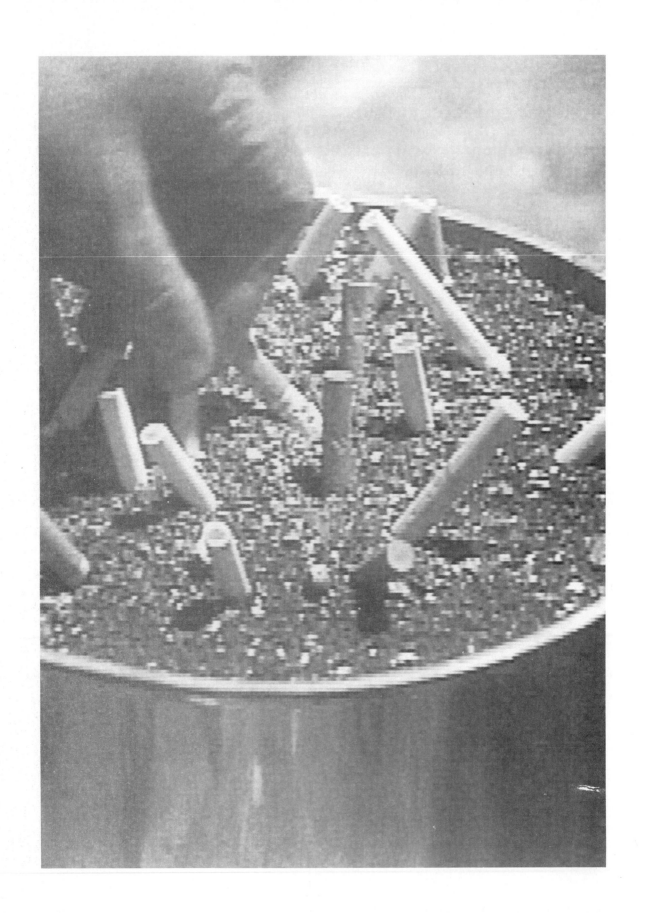

Lesson 19

Tobacco

If you can't breathe, nothing else matters.

American Lung Association

Overview

There is absolutely no doubt that tobacco causes the most preventable illness in the United States today. Though tobacco advertisements still portray smoking as glamorous or macho, there is nothing glamorous or macho about the damage that tobacco does to the body. Death from the tobacco-related lung diseases is long and agonizing, with the patient gasping for each breath. The advertisements don't mention that, or the other problems associated with tobacco. Of particular concern is the effect of tobacco on children. From the problems caused in the unborn child to the increase in respiratory diseases experienced by the children of smoking parents, the effects of tobacco affect the innocent. Lung disease is the fourth most common cause of death in the United States today.

The factors that cause people to start smoking and continue to smoke are varied, but of interest is the fact that most smokers would rather be non-smokers. The addiction properties of nicotine are very strong indeed. This physical need added to the psychological one makes it very difficult to stop smoking. Fortunately, through education and a more health-conscious society, fewer people are starting to smoke. Efforts by the American Lung Association and other groups concerned with the effects of passive smoking have also caused legislation prohibiting smoking in many areas, an important step in lowering the risk to non-smokers.

Though we probably will not reach the goal of a smoke-free society by the year 2000, there are signs of hope that at some point in the future we will be able to study tobacco from a historical perspective rather than having to contend with it as a major health threat. In the meantime, if we can persuade our young people not to begin to smoke, we will be much closer to a truly healthy society.

Learning Objectives

Goal: You should be able to discuss the significance of tobacco use, the health consequences of tobacco use for the smoker and non-smoker, and ways in which the problems associated with tobacco use are being combatted.

Objectives: Upon completion of this lesson, you should be able to:

1. Discuss the history of tobacco use, tobacco advertising, and the various factors that influence tobacco use.

2. Describe the major substances in tobacco and tobacco smoke, their effects on the body, the relationship of tobacco use and various major diseases, and the effects of tobacco on the lives of others.

3. Discuss the various types of programs that help people stop smoking and positive alternatives to tobacco use.

Study Assignments

Pay careful attention to the following assignments. The chapter number may not be the same as the lesson number.

Textbook: Chapter 15, "Tobacco," pp. 388-405

Video: "Tobacco"

Key Terms

Watch for these terms and pay particular attention to what each one means, as you follow the textbook and video.

Nicotine	**Emphysema**
Tar	**Passive/second-hand smoking**
Benzopyrene	**Hypoarousal**
Bronchitis	

Text Focus Points

Before you read the textbook assignment, review the following points to help focus your thoughts. After you complete the assignment, write out your responses to reinforce what you have learned.

1. Discuss the history of tobacco use in this country. Include the role of tobacco advertising.

2. Describe the major substances in tobacco and tobacco smoke and the effects on the body.

3. What is the relationship of tobacco use to the various major diseases? Be specific.

4. How does tobacco use affect the lives of others including the unborn child?

5. Explain the various factors that influence tobacco use including physiological and psychological dependence.

6. Identify and describe some of the types of programs designed to help people stop smoking. Include some positive alternatives to tobacco use.

Experts Interviewed

In the video segment of this lesson, the following medical and health professionals share their expertise to help you understand the material presented.

Jacqueline C. Flowers, M.P.H., M.Ed., Board of Directors, American Lung Association, New York, New York

Gary Harris, M.D., Professor and Interim Chair, Department of Medicine, The University of Texas Health Science Center, San Antonio, Texas

Video Focus Points

The following questions are designed to help you get the most from the video segment of this lesson. Review them before you watch the video. After viewing the video segment, write responses to reinforce what you have learned.

1. Explain some of the social, psychological, and physiological factors that influence tobacco use.

2. Describe the effects of smoking on the non-smoker, including the unborn child and children of smokers.

3. How does the tobacco industry attempt to replace smokers, particularly with women, minorities, and teenagers.

4. Describe some of the benefits of giving up smoking and the importance of not beginning to smoke.

Individual Health Plan

This portion of the lesson is designed to enable you to apply the information you have learned to your own life situation and improve the quality of your life. You should do any exercise assigned, complete the journal portion of the plan, then put this portion of the health plan into practice in your life.

If you are a smoker, complete the self-assessment on pages 402 and 403 in your textbook. Using the information you have gained, write a stop smoking plan for yourself in your journal. Now, carry out your plan. If you need additional help contact the American Lung Association or American Cancer Society in your area.

If you are a non-smoker, list in your journal the times in your day that you are exposed to passive smoking. Plan ways in which you could reduce this exposure. Take action on your plan.

Enrichment Opportunities

These suggestions guide you if you want more information on this lesson, want to explore new ideas, or if your instructor requires it. If you are doing this section as a course requirement, consult with your instructor for specific guidelines or directions.

1. If you have a friend or loved one who smokes, interview them and find out why they smoke, why it is hard for them to quit, and how they have tried to quit. See if there are ways that you might help them become non-smokers if they want to.

2. Contact the American Lung Association, American Cancer Society, and/or the American Heart Association in your area and find out more about their programs related to tobacco use.

3. Find out about the Clean Indoor Air legislation that exists in your community. If none exists or if you don't think it is adequate, get involved with some of the groups trying to improve the quality of indoor air.

Practice Test

After reading the assignment and watching the video, you should be able to answer the Practice Test questions. Tests also include essay questions that are similar to the Text Focus Points, the Video Focus Points, and the Objectives. When you have completed the Practice Test questions, turn to the Answer Key to score your answers.

1. Tobacco first became an important cash crop
   A   during colonial days
   B.   during the American revolution.
   C.   after the civil war.
   D.   after the turn of the century.

2. The intake of nicotine leads to feelings of increased
   A.   anxiety.
   B.   alertness.
   C.   depression.
   D.   stress.

3. Which of the following diseases has NOT been associated with the use of tobacco?
   A.   Atherosclerosis
   B.   Heart disease
   C.   Bladder cancer
   D.   Herpes

4. Because of the potential damage to their children, pregnant women are advised to
   A.   use only smokeless tobacco during pregnancy.
   B   cut down to less than a pack a day during pregnancy.
   C.   smoke only in the first trimester of a pregnancy.
   D.   stop the use of tobacco completely during pregnancy.

5. The reason that most people start smoking is
   A.   relaxation.
   B.   social pressure.
   C.   stimulation.
   D.   taste.

6. Substitution of a healthy activity for smoking at certain times is used in
   A.   behavior modification.
   B.   individual programs.
   C.   group programs.
   D.   professional therapy.

7. One of the reasons that people continue to smoke is that nicotine is
   A. addicting.
   B. pleasurable.
   C. relatively harmless.
   D. carcinogenic.

8. Tobacco use by the pregnant woman can
   A. produce little damage in the fetus.
   B. result in a more difficult labor.
   C. seriously affect the fetus.
   D. cause liver failure in the fetus.

9. The tobacco industry attempts to appeal to women and minorities by portraying smoking as all the following EXCEPT as
   A. reality.
   B. sophisticated.
   C. healthy.
   D. sexy.

10. One of the main functions of smoking cessation group programs is that members receive
    A. guaranteed results.
    B. support from each other.
    C. in-depth psychotherapy.
    D. medication.

11. The surgeon general recently reported that tobacco use is the cause of death in our society that is most _____.

12. The carbon monoxide found in tobacco smoke impairs the blood's capacity to carry _____.

13. Marked by coughing and difficulty breathing, inflammation of the epithelium leads to chronic _____.

14. When a person is physically dependent on a drug like tobacco, the condition is termed _____.

True or False
15. Carbon monoxide, a gas in tobacco smoke, impairs the body's capacity to carry oxygen.

16. Though it is suspected that smoking is related to cancer, the positive evidence is still lacking.

17. There is evidence that young female smokers are influenced by boyfriends and husbands who smoke.

18. Group programs such as those sponsored by the American Lung Association use lectures, films, discussions, and practical tips in the effort to help people stop smoking.

19. Babies born of mothers who smoke are frequently low in birth weight and experience other health problems.

20. The nicotine patch guarantees that the smoker will be able to stop smoking.

Answer Key

These are the correct answers with reference to the Learning Objectives, and to the source of the information: the Textbook Focus Points, Levy, *et al. Life and Health,* and the Video Focus Points. Page numbers are also given for the Textbook Focus Points. "KT" indicates questions with Key Terms defined.

Question	Answer	Learning Objective	Textbook Focus Point (page no.)		Video Focus Point
1.	A	19.1	1 (p. 389)		
2.	B	19.2	2 (p. 391)		
3.	D	19.2	3 (p. 393)		
4.	D	19.2	4 (p. 396)		
5.	B	19.1	5 (p. 397)		
6.	A	19.3	6 (pp. 401-402)		
7.	A	19.1			1
8.	C	19.2			2
9.	A	19.1			3
10.	B	19.3			4
11.	preventable	19.1	1 (p. 389)		
12.	oxygen	19.2	2 (p. 392)	KT	
13.	bronchitis	19.2	3 (p. 394)	KT	
14.	addiction	19.1			1
15.	T	19.2	2 (p. 392)	KT	
16.	F	19.2	3 (p. 395)		
17.	T	19.1	5 (p. 399)		
18.	T	19.3	6 (p. 401)		
19.	T	19.2			2
20.	F	19.3			4

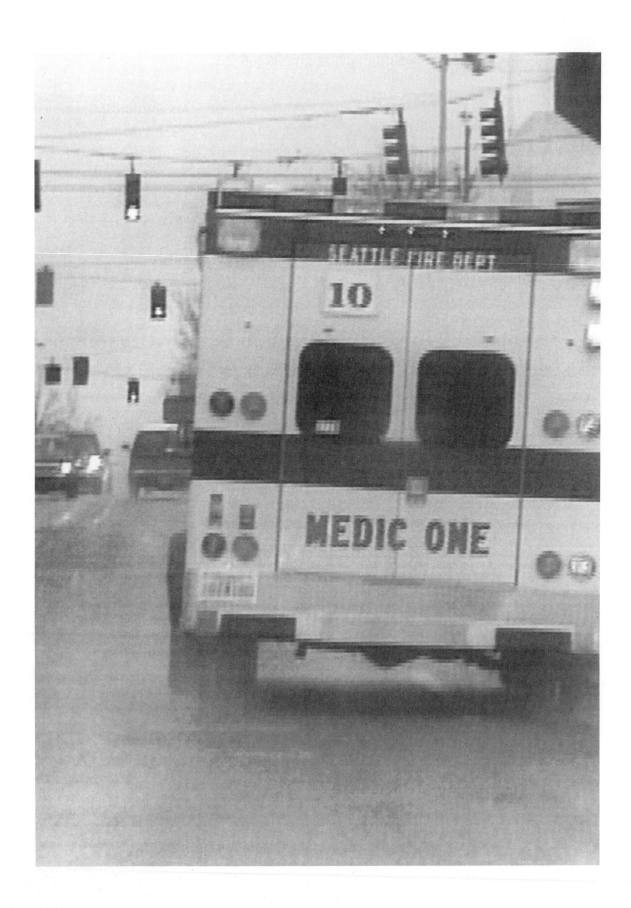

Lesson 20

Injury Prevention

I can tell you from my perspective as a physician, seeing the tragedies of young people coming into our trauma centers with their severe injuries, multiple fractures, brain injury . . . I look upon the fact that these are tragedies that could have been prevented, or if not entirely prevented, could be greatly reduced.

Louis Sullivan, M.D.

Overview

We often hear the expression, "It was an accident." In reality, there is no such thing as a true accident. If we begin with the "accident" and work backward, we will always find that if some aspect had happened differently, if a different decision had been made, the outcome would have changed. This concept becomes very important as we look at how injuries most often happen and who is at risk. This lesson also becomes very important when we consider that virtually everyone of us will sustain at least one injury in our life (usually quite a few) and that injuries are the leading cause of death from birth to age 45.

Consider the fact that most often your own decision and subsequent action either causes or prevents the incident that leads to injury. If you approach your life with this bit of knowledge, you will be likely to make decisions that reduce your risk for injury. You have heard the expression "driving defensively." Expand this concept to "living defensively."

The other very important part of living a healthy lifestyle is knowing what to do when injury does occur. Each year many lives could be saved and serious injuries prevented if more people knew basic first aid and cardiopulmonary resuscitation (CPR). Many of us have seen the panic that frequently surrounds an emergency situation. Panic inevitably results when people do not know what to do. Spending the short time it takes to learn first aid and CPR makes the difference in knowing what to do. Remember, the life you save may be your own or that of your loved one.

A very important part of the decisions we make to achieve a healthy lifestyle include those that will decrease our risk of injury, as well as giving us the knowledge to function effectively if injury does happen.

Learning Objectives

Goal: You should be able to explain reasons injuries happen, types of injuries most frequent in various situations, principles of injury prevention, and basic principles of emergency care.

Objectives: Upon completion of this lesson, you should be able to:

1. Explain why injuries happen, discuss the threshold theory, and the agent-host-environment model, and describe the role that violence plays in causing injuries.

2. Describe the types of injuries that occur most frequently at home, at work, and during recreation. Discuss the individuals most at risk for injuries with each and the factors associated with motor vehicle injuries, falls, burns, drownings, poisonings, and violence-related injuries.

3. Explain how injury prevention is related to the agent-host-environment model, the two major approaches to accident prevention, active and passive prevention, and the effectiveness of each.

4. List the basic principles of emergency care and explain the emergency treatment of stopped breathing, choking, burns, and drowning.

Study Assignments

Pay careful attention to the following assignments. The chapter number may not be the same as the lesson number.

Textbook: Chapter 16, "Injuries and Their Prevention," pp. 406-432

Video: "Accidents and Injury Prevention"

Key Terms

Watch for these terms and pay particular attention to what each one means, as you follow the textbook and video.

Kinetic energy	CPR
Thermal energy	Heimlich maneuver
Chemical energy	Shock
Electrical energy	Direct pressure
Radiation energy	Pressure points
Vector	Thermal burn
Violence	Chemical burn
Intentional injuries	First-degree burns
Active prevention	Second-degree burns
Passive prevention	Third-degree burns

Textbook Focus Points

Before you read the textbook assignment, review the following points to help focus your thoughts. After you complete the assignment, write out your responses to reinforce what you have learned.

1. Why do injuries happen? Include the threshold theory and the agent-host-environment model in your discussion.

2. Identify some of the most common types of injuries that occur at home and those at highest risk for home injuries. What are ways of preventing home injuries?

3. What kinds of injuries are most common at work? Who is most often affected?

4. Discuss the most common recreational injuries and the sports most related to serious injury.

5. Describe the role that violence plays in causing injuries.

6. Identify and discuss the factors associated with motor vehicle injuries, falls, burns, drownings, poisonings, and violence-related injuries.

---

7. Define active and passive prevention, identify several active and passive preventive measures, and discuss their effectiveness. Include individual strategies for injury prevention.

8. List the basic principles of emergency care and describe the emergency care needed for stopped breathing, choking, burns, shock, and drowning.

Experts Interviewed

In the video segment of this lesson, the following medical and health professionals share their expertise to help you understand the material presented.

Richard A. Schieber, M.D., Medical Epidemiologist, Centers for Disease Control and Prevention, Atlanta, Georgia

Gary R. Strand, Chief, Medic One Program, Seattle Fire Department, Seattle, Washington

Richard A. Newbrey, Lieutenant, Medical Services Officer, Medic One Program, Seattle Fire Department, Seattle, Washington

Louis W. Sullivan, M.D., President, Morehouse School of Medicine, Atlanta, Georgia, Former Secretary, U.S. Department of Health and Human Services

Video Focus Points

The following questions are designed to help you get the most from the video segment of this lesson. Review them before you watch the video. After viewing the video segment, write responses to reinforce what you have learned.

1. Discuss the various factors involved in causing accidents and injury. Explain accidents in terms of the agent-host-environment model.

2. Describe safety measures that reduce the risk of injury at home and on the street. Why is taking responsibility for one's own safety so important?

3. Explain the importance of first aid and cardiopulmonary resuscitation in reducing severity of injury or illness.

4. How can individuals reduce their own risk of injury related to violence?

Individual Health Plan

This portion of the lesson is designed to enable you to apply the information you have learned to your own life situation and improve the quality of your life. You should do any exercise assigned, complete the journal portion of the plan, then put this portion of the health plan into practice in your life.

> Complete the Self-Assessment on page 409 of your textbook. Use this as a basis to examine the level of risk for injury in your own lifestyle. In your journal write an evaluation of your own risks for injury in the various aspects of your life. Develop a written plan of action to lower your risk of injury. If you have not already learned first aid and CPR, include this in your plan. Develop a time-line for taking action on your plan.

Enrichment Opportunities

These suggestions guide you if you want more information on this lesson, want to explore new ideas, or if your instructor requires it. If you are doing this section as a course requirement, consult with your instructor for specific guidelines or directions.

1. Interview a paramedic, an emergency care physician, or nurse, and discuss the types of injuries they most often treat, and the types of individuals most often involved.

2. Interview a police officer and learn his or her perspective regarding the role violence and alcohol play in injuries.

Practice Test

After reading the assignment and watching the video, you should be able to answer the Practice Test questions. Tests also include essay questions that are similar to the Text Focus Points, the Video Focus Points, and the Objectives. When you have completed the Practice Test questions, turn to the Answer Key to score your answers.

1. According to the threshold theory, injury occurs when energy exceeds the
   A. output an individual provides.
   B. body's rate of metabolism.
   C. limit of a person's skills and capabilities.
   D. total amount of energy required to gain momentum.

2. Placing toxic substances within the reach of children is an example of creating a dangerous
   A. host factor.
   B. environment.
   C. agent.
   D. accident.

3. Now recognized as one of the nation's most dangerous industries is
   A. manufacturing.
   B. agriculture.
   C. medicine.
   D. aviation.

4. In which of the following types of sports is an injury most likely to occur?
   A. Noncontact sports
   B. Noncompetitive sports
   C. Contact sports
   D. Sports that involve running

5. Injuries caused by interpersonal violence such as homicide and assault are sometimes classified as
   A. nonviolent injuries.
   B. planned injuries.
   C. accidental injuries.
   D. intentional injuries.

6. Studies show that motor vehicle crashes in which alcohol plays a role tend to be
   A. more severe than other crashes.
   B. less severe than other crashes.
   C. less common than other crashes.
   D. less fatal than other crashes.

7. Which of the following measures requires active prevention to be useful?
   A. Automatic seat belts
   B. Improved street lighting
   C. Safety switches on power tools
   D. Bicycle helmets

8. What is the first goal of emergency care?
   A. Stop bleeding
   B. Close wounds
   C. Prevent further injury
   D. Get the victim to lie down

9. The agent factor in a motorcycle accident is
   A. crowded streets.
   B. careless drivers.
   C. rainy weather.
   D. energy of the motorcycle.

10. When riding a motorcycle or a bicycle, it is important to
    A. choose an expensive bike.
    B. wear protective gear.
    C. use the left lane.
    D. avoid freeways.

11. An emergency can be defined as
    A. a major accident.
    B. a stoppage of breathing.
    C. a heart attack.
    D. an event the individual cannot cope with.

12. A good defense against a perpetrator is to
    A. do the unexpected.
    B. carry a firearm.
    C. fight the perpetrator.
    D. call "help."

13. A shock caused by a short circuit in a plug-in appliance is an example of the type of energy termed _____.

14. The type of prevention that requires little or no individual action on the part of those being protected is characterized as _____.

15. The type of pressure applied to a wound to keep it from bleeding is called _____.

16. The blood alcohol level of the driver of a car is considered the _____.

True or False
17. In applying the agent-host environment model to motor vehicle accidents, the automobile would be considered the vector.

18. While clothing related burns are still fairly common in children, improved flammability standards for children's clothes have resulted in a decreased risk.

19. Most houses have adequate safety measures built into them.

20. First aid and cardiopulmonary resuscitation are complicated procedures best left to paramedics and other professionals.

Answer Key

These are the correct answers with reference to the Learning Objectives, and to the source of the information: the Textbook Focus Points, Levy, *et al. Life and Health,* and the Video Focus Points. Page numbers are also given for the Textbook Focus Points. KT indicates questions with Key Terms defined.

Question	Answer	Learning Objective	Textbook Focus Point (page no.)	Video Focus Point
1.	C	20.1	1 (p. 408)	
2.	B	20.2	2 (pp. 411-412)	
3.	B	20.2	3 (p. 412)	
4.	C	20.2	4 (p. 413)	
5.	D	20.1	5 (p. 413) KT	
6.	A	20.2	6 (p. 414)	
7.	D	20.3	7 (p. 419)	
8.	C	20.4	8 (p. 424)	
9.	D	20.1		1
10.	B	20.3		2
11.	D	20.3		3
12.	A	20.1		4
13.	electrical	20.1	1 (p. 408) KT	
14.	passive	20.3	7 (p. 420) KT	
15.	direct	20.4	8 (p. 427) KT	
16.	host	20.1		1
17.	T	20.1	1 (p. 410) KT	
18.	T	20.2	6 (p. 415)	
19.	F	20.3		2
20.	F	20.3		3

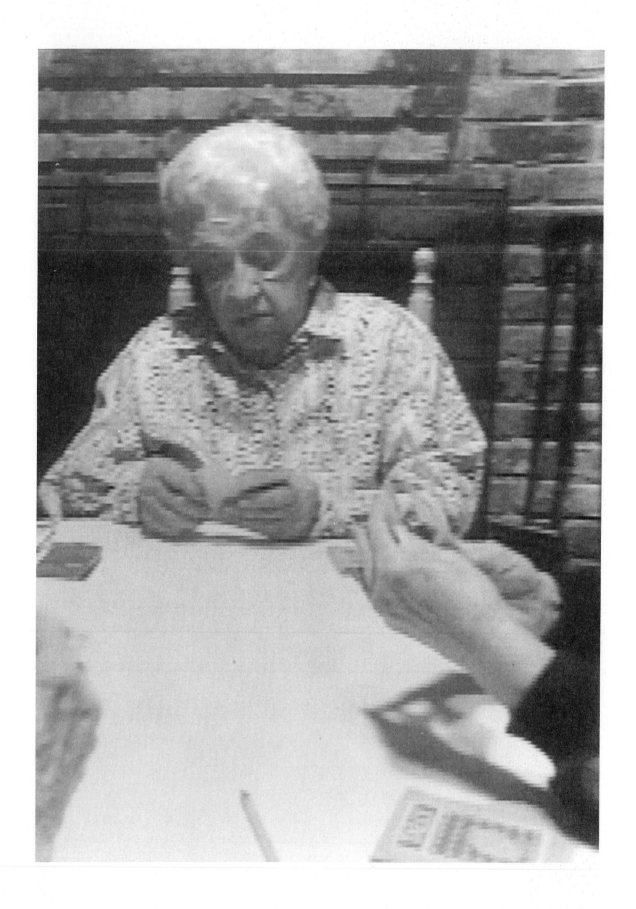

Lesson 21

Aging

So often when you get to this age, people seem to think you're supposed to run around with people your age and they want to categorize you. ... There is no reason at all to enjoy people your own age just because they are your own age because age covers the entire spectrum of society.

Ellen Mallum

Overview

How do you feel about getting older? Really? What is your image of what it is like to age? Intellectually you may be able to accept the idea that we all are aging. Emotionally it may be a different story. If we see being older as being feeble and frail, we may have very strong negative feelings. If we have come to terms with the fact that aging is a normal process that we all share, we will be able to find the "golden" in the golden years.

Though we may think of aging as a time of frailty, nursing home care, and dependency on others, this is the picture of only a few of our aging population. In reality, most older people are living independently and enjoying active, productive lives. Though the older person is at higher risk for certain types of illnesses and injuries, these are by no means inevitable. Much of the quality of our later years is determined by the decisions we make and the lifestyle we live in our earlier years. If we learn to care for our health and develop a healthy lifestyle throughout the earlier part of our lives, we are very likely to continue this into our later years, thus improving the quality of our later life.

The concept of aging with dignity is a very important one. If we talk to older people, the thing that means the most to them is maintaining their independence and control over their own destiny — in other words, their dignity. It is important that we keep this in mind as we relate to our aging relatives and friends. We know that good psychosocial support systems and healthy lifestyles are keys to the well-being of the older person. The more we help insure that they maintain as much independence as possible, the higher the quality of life they will enjoy.

As we make our own life choices and decisions, we also want to remember how very important these will be to our own chances of aging with dignity and good health. Each of us has significant control over our own destiny — it is up to us to make wise lifestyle choices that will guide us toward the quality of life that we desire.

Learning Objectives

Goal: You should be able to compare normal aging with pathological aging, discuss Erickson's stages of growth and development, theories of aging, illnesses and injuries most common in the elderly, and ways that individuals maintain their health as they age.

Objectives: Upon completion of this lesson, you should be able to:

1. Compare normal aging with pathological aging, discuss Erickson's stages of growth and development, the four theories of aging based on genetic and physiologic factors, and discuss the changes in appearance, body tissue, and body functions that occur with aging.

2. Discuss the diseases and injuries most common in the elderly, including Alzheimer's disease and suicide, and why the elderly are more prone to illness and injury.

3. Explain ways in which individuals maintain their physical, emotional, intellectual, social, and spiritual health as they grow older, and how individuals can help improve the life and health of their aging family members, friends, children, and future generations.

Study Assignments

Pay careful attention to the following assignments. The chapter number may not be the same as the lesson number.

Textbook: Chapter 17, "Lifestyle and Growing Older", pp. 434-457

Video: "Aging"

Key Terms

Watch for these terms and pay particular attention to what each one means, as you follow the textbook and video.

Aging	Diabetes
Normal aging	Arthritis
Pathological aging	Alzheimer's disease
Gerontology	Cellular aging
Life span	Genetic limits
Life expectancy	Error theory
Fluid intelligence	Free radical theory
Crystallized intelligence	Somatic mutation theory
Osteoporosis	Cross-linkage theory

Text Focus Points

Before you read the textbook assignment, review the following points to help focus your thoughts. After you complete the assignment, write out your responses to reinforce what you have learned.

1. Why are people afraid of the aging process? What are the differences in normal aging and pathological aging? Include explanation of life span and life expectancy.

2. Describe how people change as they age. Identify and discuss Erickson's stages of growth and development in a person's life.

3. What changes in appearance, body tissue, and body functions occur during aging, and why do these happen?

4. Distinguish between fluid intelligence and crystallized intelligence and explain how cognitive functions change as a person grows older.

5. Why are the elderly more susceptible to injury and infectious disease than the general population? How can the risk of having accidents be minimized?

---

6. Identify the most common chronic diseases that affect the elderly. Describe disability and explain the effects of arthritis on disability.

7. Discuss the effects of Alzheimer's disease and the incidence of depression and suicide among the elderly.

8. Discuss the causes and theories of aging.

9. How can individuals maintain their physical, emotional, intellectual, social, and spiritual health as they grow older?

10. How can individuals help improve the life and health of their aging family members and friends, their children, and future generations?

Experts Interviewed

In the video segment of this lesson, the following health professionals share their expertise to help you understand the material presented.

William J. Evans, Ph.D., Chief, Human Physiology Laboratory, USDA Human Nutrition Research Center on Aging,Tufts University, Boston, Massachusetts

Charles S. Wolfe, M.A., Ed.S., Consultant and Lecturer, Charles S. Wolfe and Associates, Inc., Aventura, Florida

Video Focus Points

The following questions are designed to help you get the most from the video segment of this lesson. Review them before you watch the video. After viewing the video segment, write responses to reinforce what you have learned.

1. Describe some of the body changes that occur with aging and why these occur.

2. Explain the psychosocial stages from infancy to old age described by Erickson.

---

3. What are some of the ways that we can increase our health and the quality of our life as we grow older. Include things that we can do to improve the quality of life of our older relatives and friends.

Individual Health Plan

This portion of the lesson is designed to enable you to apply the information you have learned to your own life situation and improve the quality of your life. You should do any exercise assigned, complete the journal portion of the plan, then put this portion of the health plan into practice in your life.

Think about the important older people in your life, the quality of their life and your relationships with them. Based on what you have learned in this lesson, how would you evaluate these things? Consider the lifestyle you are leading and the planning (or lack of it) that you are doing for your own later years. In your journal, develop some plans for your life designed to help insure that you have the opportunity to age with dignity. If there are things that you would like to do differently in your relationships with the important older people in your life, include those. Now begin to carry out these plans.

Enrichment Opportunities

These suggestions guide you if you want more information on this lesson, want to explore new ideas, or if your instructor requires it. If you are doing this section as a course requirement, consult with your instructor for specific guidelines or directions.

1. Arrange an interview with a gerontologist, geriatric nurse, or other professional who works with senior citizens and discuss the life of senior citizens including their special needs and problems.

2. Visit an older person living in a nursing home and one living independently. Compare their lifestyle, health, feelings, problems, and quality of their lives.

Practice Test

After reading the assignment and watching the video, you should be able to answer the Practice Test questions. Tests also include essay questions that are similar to the Text Focus Points, the Video Focus Points, and the Objectives. When you have completed the Practice Test questions, turn to the Answer Key to score your answers.

1. Many people fear the aging process because they believe that
   A. physical and mental decline is inevitable.
   B. aging reflects destructive health habits.
   C. chronological age is a good predictor of mental health status.
   D. experiences of being old cannot be improved.

2. Which of the following has NOT been shown to be associated with high levels of physical function in old age?
   A. Absence of hypertension
   B. Sedentary lifestyle
   C. History of never smoking
   D. Maintenance of normal weight

3. Which of the following is NOT a true statement about aging?
   A. Appearance changes.
   B. Negative attitudes grow.
   C. Bodily functions deteriorate.
   D. Susceptibility to injury increases.

4. It is recommended that older people receive preventive immunizations because they
   A. often eat food contaminated by bacteria.
   B. are more prone to have accidents.
   C. may be less attentive to body cleanliness.
   D. have less resistance to disease-producing organisms.

5. Which should NOT be encouraged for as long as possible in people who suffer from Alzheimer's disease?
   A. Maintaining daily routines
   B. Continuing social contacts
   C. Using medication to relieve some symptoms
   D. Increasing dependence on relatives

---

6. A person who exercises and has good diet and nutrition habits is maintaining his or her
   A. emotional health.
   B. intellectual health.
   C. physical health.
   D. social health.

7. The special influence that elderly persons can have on children does NOT include
   A. teaching them respect for others.
   B. providing support for children experiencing tension with parents.
   C. imparting their wisdom and experience
   D. providing them with gifts or spending money.

8. The aspect of normal aging over which people have most control is
   A. change of visual acuity.
   B. level of fitness.
   C. density of bones.
   D. elasticity of skin.

9. According to Erikson, the period of life when parenting responsibilities decrease and people begin assessing their career achievements is known as
   A. young adulthood.
   B. middle age.
   C. older adulthood.
   D. old age.

10. Supports that insure a higher quality of life in the later years are LEAST likely to include
    A. family and friends.
    B. quality of health.
    C. specific religious denomination.
    D. leisure and pleasure activities.

11. Many people have married or established lifelong commitment by the time they enter _____.

12. If an individual has the ability to use accumulated knowledge and learning, he or she has _____.

13. That cells introduce and compound errors in the genetic material as they divide is part of the _____.

14. The time when one's children are grown and some outward signs of aging are beginning to occur is termed _____.

True or False

15. Because of varied environments and lifestyles, life expectancy differs significantly among different groups within the population.

16. Most elderly can perform personal-care activities and other activities of daily living.

17. Physical well-being and intellectual and emotional health seem unrelated among the elderly.

18. The aging process begins at about age 55.

19. In old age, social relationships, sporting activities, and hobbies are begun as the new focus of life.

20. Lifestyle choices in early life greatly affect health in the later years.

Answer Key

These are the correct answers with reference to the Learning Objectives, and to the source of the information: the Textbook Focus Points, Levy, *et al. Life and Health,* and the Video Focus Points. Page numbers are also given for the Textbook Focus Points. "KT" indicates questions with Key Terms defined.

Question	Answer	Learning Objective	Textbook Focus Point (page no.)	Video Focus Point
1.	A	21.1	1 (p. 435)	
2	B	21.1	1 (p. 436)	
3	B	21.1	3 (pp. 440-444)	
4	D	21.2	5 (p. 444)	
5	D	21.2	7 (p. 447)	
6	C	21.3	9 (p. 450)	
7	D	21.3	10 (p. 453)	
8	B	21.1		1
9	B	21.1		2
10	C	21.3		3
11.	young adulthood	21.1	2 (p. 438)	
12.	crystallized intelligence	21.1	4 (p. 442)	KT
13.	error theory	21.1	8 (p. 449)	KT
14.	middle age	21.1		2
15	T	21.1	1 (p. 436)	
16	T	21.2	6 (p. 445)	
17	F	21.3	9 (p. 451)	
18	F	21.1		1
19	F	21.1		2
20	T	21.3		3

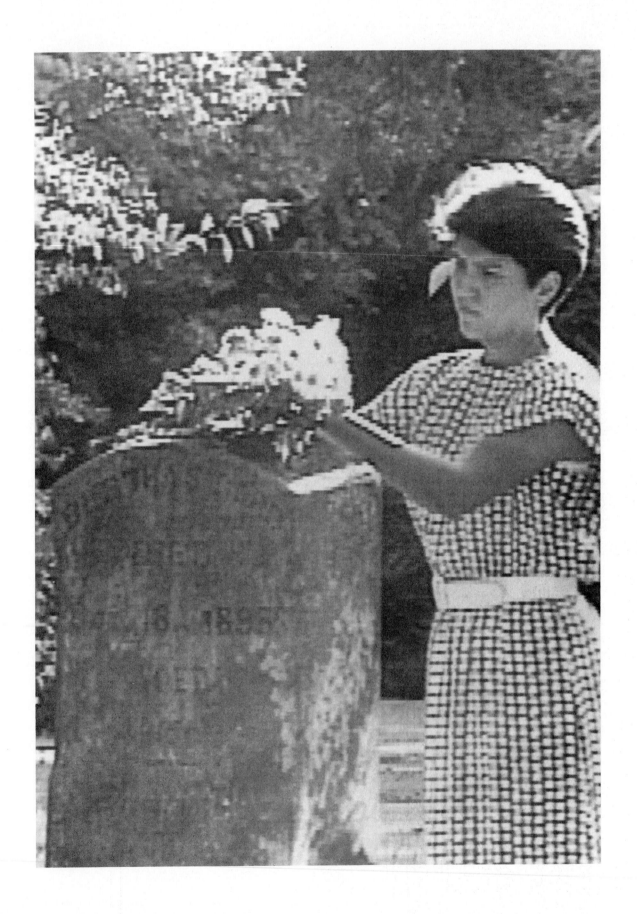

Lesson 22

Death and Dying

When I think about what gives me the strength to look at dying and not be afraid, I realize that the strength giving element in my life did not occur two years ago or three years ago; it's not related to the cancer. It's really related to whatever the tenure of my life has been and it's not changed dramatically and I'm okay with the fact that I was born, I lived a good life, and I'm dying.

Mary Stupp

Overview

Elisabeth Kübler-Ross called death "the final stage of growth." My friend, Mary, talked of "my last great adventure." Others speak of the "angel of death." What does death mean to you? Have you come to the acceptance of your own mortality and that of your loved ones? If these questions frighten you or make you uneasy, you are not alone. Many share your fears and uncertainty.

No one really knows what dying is. Many have had similar "near death" experiences, which have given us a glimpse, but no one actually knows. What we do know is that each of us will experience death, and death is a normal part of the human experience.

The way in which we support dying loved ones and even accept our own mortality depends largely on our own feelings about death and dying. It is important that we understand the process, are able to think about it and to talk about it.

Acceptance of death certainly does not come all at once, and coping with the death of a loved one is not an easy process. Elisabeth Kübler-Ross described stages that one may go through in accepting death. However she also says that people do not go neatly through these stages and some never get to the stage of acceptance. Most experts feel that we generally die in much the same manner as we have lived. In other words, if we have led a fairly centered, healthy life, we will be able to accept the idea of death. Our emotional hardiness allows us to cope with the experience of life and death.

All too often our own fears and conflicts make it difficult or impossible to offer support to the very ones we love the most at the time that they need us. Some of us cannot bear to even visit the dying, much less talk of their feelings and thoughts. It is as though if we don't acknowledge death, it will not happen. Dying patients need to talk. They need us to be able to listen and share feelings with them.

An important part of our health is to be able to also accept the concept of dying and death. If we can be at peace with this final stage of growth, our life will be much fuller, much more meaningful.

Learning Objectives

Goal: You should be able to discuss differing views of death, the stages of acceptance of death, and the grieving process.

Objectives: Upon completion of this lesson, you should be able to:

1. Describe measures of death and discuss some typical responses to death of children, adults, and the elderly.

2. Discuss the stages of acceptance of death developed by Elisabeth Kübler-Ross, the factors that affect a person's attitudes about death, responses expressed by dying patients as death approaches, the role of the will to live and suicide.

3. Discuss the care of the dying, and the goals and advantages of hospice care.

4. Discuss the making of a will, the categories of euthanasia and the legal, ethical, and moral issues involved.

5. Discuss the purpose of funerals and differing funeral customs, the stages of the mourning process, the patterns of bereavement, and how people can cope with grief.

Study Assignment

Pay careful attention to the following assignments. The chapter number may not be the same as the lesson number.

Textbook: Chapter 18, "Dying and Death", pp. 458-481

Video: "Death and Dying"

Key Terms

Watch for these terms and pay particular attention to what each one means, as you follow the textbook and video.

Thanatology	**Passive euthanasia**
Clinical death	**Active euthanasia**
Brain death	***Quinlan*** and ***Saikewicz*** **cases**
Social death	**Living will**
Hospice	**"Natural death" laws**
Will	**Mourning**
Executor	**Bereavement**
Donor card	**Grief**
Euthanasia	**"Normal" grief**

Text Focus Points

Before you read the textbook assignment, review the following points to help focus your thoughts. After you complete the assignment, write out your responses to reinforce what you have learned.

1. Define thanatology. Distinguish between clinical death and brain death as final measures of death.

2. Describe social death. Express some of the typical responses to death by children, adults, and the elderly.

3. Identify and discuss the stages of acceptance of death developed by Elisabeth Kübler-Ross. What emotional needs do dying people have?

4. Describe several responses expressed by dying patients as death approaches.

---

5. What role does the will to live play in the dying process? Why do people attempt or commit suicide and what factors contribute to suicide?

6. Identify the goals of hospice care including the advantages of hospice care and home care over hospital and nursing home care.

7. Identify the critical issues to consider in preparing for death. Discuss the importance of making a will. What is the function of an executor? What is a donor card?

8. List the categories of euthanasia and discuss the legal precedents involved.

9. What purpose do funerals serve? Describe some of the stages that people experience in the mourning or grieving process.

10. Discuss several different patterns of bereavement that people may experience including that of children and of parents.

11. How can people cope with the grief of losing a loved one?

Expert Interviewed

In the video segment of this lesson, the following medical professional shares her expertise to help you understand the material presented.

Elisabeth Kübler-Ross, M.D., President, Elisabeth Kübler-Ross Center, Head Waters, Virginia

Video Focus Points

The following questions are designed to help you get the most from the video segment of this lesson. Review them before you watch the video. After viewing the video segment, write responses to reinforce what you have learned.

1. Explain the five stages of acceptance of death described by Elisabeth Kübler-Ross.

2. How can family and friends offer the dying patient emotional support?

3. Why is the grieving process important? Do all people grieve in the same way?

Individual Health Plan

This portion of the lesson is designed to enable you to apply the information you have learned to your own life situation and improve the quality of your life. You should do any exercise assigned, complete the journal portion of the plan, then put this portion of the health plan into practice in your life.

In your journal, describe the feelings about death and dying you had before this lesson. Complete the Self-Assessment on page 463 of your text. Did any of the answers surprise you? Record the thoughts and feelings that you have now that you have completed this lesson. Has anything changed? In what way? If you find yourself very troubled about death, consider consulting a counselor or clergy member.

Enrichment Opportunities

These suggestions guide you if you want more information on this lesson, want to explore new ideas, or if your instructor requires it. If you are doing this section as a course requirement, consult with your instructor for specific guidelines or directions.

1. Contact a hospice facility and discuss hospice care.

2. Talk with health professionals, lawyers and clergy concerning issues such as organ transplants, living wills, and euthanasia.

3. Visit a funeral home and discuss funeral arrangements with a staff member.

Practice Test

After reading the assignment and watching the video, you should be able to answer the Practice Test questions. Tests also include essay questions that are similar to the Text Focus Points, the Video Focus Points, and the Objectives. When you have completed the Practice Test questions, turn to the Answer Key to score your answers.

1. The field of research on death and dying is called
   A. euthanasia.
   B. hospice.
   C. thanatology.
   D. bereavement.

2. The final days for a dying person may be made more difficult by all EXCEPT
   A. treating the dying person as if already dead.
   B. giving less medical attention to the dying person.
   C. expressing love and talking to the dying person.
   D. acting as though the dying person was incapable of making a decision.

3. A terminally ill patient who hopes to live long enough to see his or her child graduate from college is in which stage of dying?
   A. Anger
   B. Bargaining
   C. Depression
   D. Acceptance

4. Which of the following probably would help alleviate a dying person's pain?
   A. Isolation
   B. Depression
   C. Anxiety
   D. Emotional support

5. Which of the following is NOT a true statement about suicide?
   A. Suicide is a self-destructive act.
   B. Suicide is usually committed by a person who faces serious illness or disability.
   C. Suicide may result from culturally supported beliefs.
   D. Suicide is significantly influenced by heredity.

6. Several states have "natural death" laws that allow patients to refuse
   A. organ donations.
   B. treatment for terminal illnesses.
   C. to write living wills.
   D. embalming procedures.

7. Funerals are of psychological value to the survivors because they provide for all of the following EXCEPT
   A. something concrete for survivors to do.
   B. affirmation of family networks.
   C. procedure required by law.
   D. confirmation of the reality of death.

8. The way someone reacts to a death depends in part on the
   A. patterns among the bereaved.
   B. availability of memorial societies.
   C. way the loved one died.
   D. anticipatory grief structures.

9. In order to cope with death, a grieving person should NOT
   A. grow detached from the deceased.
   B. maintain supportive relationships with others.
   C. hold on to a satisfactory self-image.
   D. deny feelings of loss.

10. Though the individual may be complaining and relatively talkative, the fourth stage in the acceptance of death includes
    A. anger.
    B. bargaining.
    C. depression.
    D. acceptance.

11. In offering support to the dying, confidants should do all the following EXCEPT
    A. appear ready to listen.
    B. reassure that things will be fine.
    C. talk about death.
    D. share feelings of love and acceptance.

12. Problems develop when people
   A. express individuality in their grieving.
   B. cannot overcome their acute grief.
   C. take six months to work through grief.
   D. talk frequently about the deceased.

13. The shunning or turning away from a dying person by friends, relatives, and others may be described as _____.

14. To make the dying patient comfortable without using devices for prolonging life is the highest priority of _____.

15. After individuals recover from the shock and denial of finding that they have a terminal illness, they usually experience _____.

16. Coming to terms with the death of a loved one usually occurs during the process of _____.

True or False
17. Because home care for the dying presents few problems and saves a significant amount of money, it is preferable.

18. Even without a will, the deceased person's wishes will be followed by a caring family.

19. The depression stage is usually a very quiet one for the dying patient.

20. An important role that friends can play is to listen to whatever the dying patient wants to talk about.

Answer Key

These are the correct answers with reference to the Learning Objectives, and to the source of the information: the Textbook Focus Points, Levy, *et al. Life and Health,* and the Video Focus Points. Page numbers are also given for the Textbook Focus Points. "KT" indicates questions with Key Terms defined.

Question	Answer	Learning Objective	Textbook Focus Point (page no.)	Video Focus Point
1.	C	22.1	1 (p. 459)	KT
2.	C	22.1	2 (p. 460)	
3.	B	22.2	3 (p. 464)	
4.	D	22.2	4 (p. 465)	
5.	B	22.2	5 (p. 466)	
6.	B	22.4	8 (p. 473)	
7.	C	22.5	9 (p. 474)	
8.	C	22.5	10 (p. 475)	
9.	D	22.5	11 (p. 479)	
10.	C	22.2		1
11.	B	22.3		2
12.	B	22.5		3
13.	social death	22.1	2 (p. 460)	KT
14.	hospice	22.3	6 (p. 469)	KT
15.	anger	22.2		1
16.	grief	22.5		3
17.	F	22.3	6 (p. 470)	
18.	F	22.4	7 (p. 470)	
19.	F	22.2		1
20.	T	22.3		2

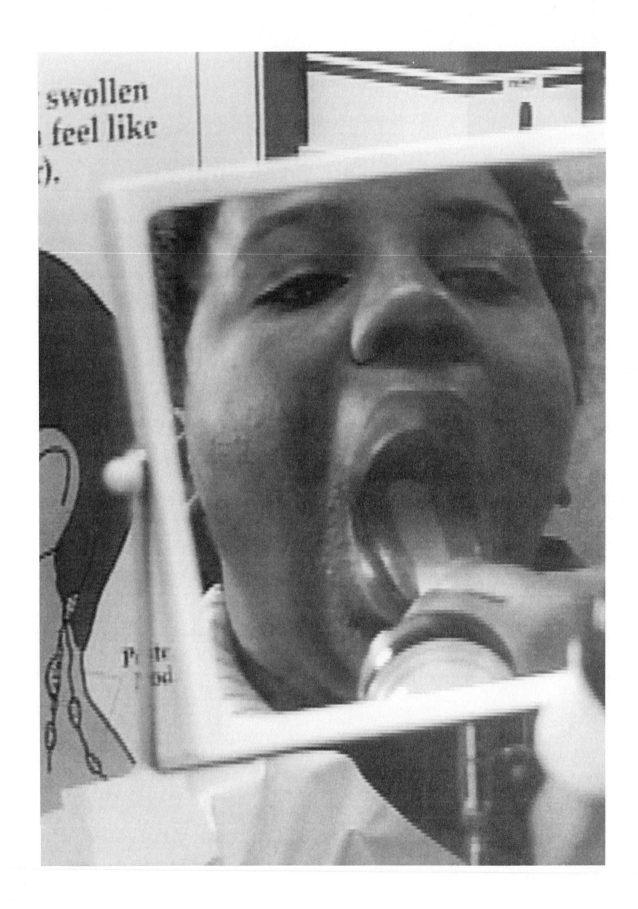

Lesson 23

Health Self-Care

Each patient carries his own doctor inside him. They come to us not knowing that truth. We are at our best when we give the doctor who resides within each patient a chance to go to work.

Albert Schweitzer, M.D.

Overview

Earlier in the history of this country, people took a great deal of responsibility for their own health care. The main reasons for this were their isolation from doctors and unavailable transportation. Then people began to rely heavily on the more accessible physicians and their newer "wonder" drugs. Now people are again realizing that they can care for many of their own minor illnesses. They have also developed more interest in some of the alternative health care methods. In a time when our health care delivery systems are overcrowded and very expensive, it is a wise person who uses good judgement in knowing when professional health care is needed and when caring for one's own minor illness is possible.

The health-activated person has adopted a lifestyle that minimizes risk of illness and injury. However, we all know that even a healthy person sometimes falls prey to a "bug" or minor injury. As we learn to listen to our body when it gives us clues that all is not well, and how to determine how serious our condition may be, we will be able to make healthy decisions about how to care for ourselves when the balance is disturbed.

Most minor illnesses are self-limiting and do not require prescription drugs. Often a simple relief of the symptoms is all the body needs to heal itself. In fact it is good to remember the old saying, "If you ignore a cold, it goes away in a week, if you treat it, it goes away in seven days." A healthy body has a remarkable amount of resiliency and ability to heal itself, if allowed. Usually all that's needed is the simplest self-care. If the symptoms don't go away, if they worsen, or if more serious signs are

---

present, it is time to get professional care. If you have doubts, call your physician's office or consult your college health center.

Through all of this remember, we have been talking about a healthy body. Once again we are reminded that we are responsible for the lifestyle that insures that our health is optimal. We can't delegate this responsibility to anyone else, not even our physician.

Learning Objectives

Goal: You should be able to explain the importance of being health-activated, the importance of physical examinations and other health measurements, and some components of the home medicine chest.

Objectives: Upon completion of this lesson, you should be able to:

1. Discuss current trends in health responsibility, the importance of being health-activated, and some of the characteristics of the health-activated person.

2. Identify some of the body's "norms," the factors that may cause them to vary, discuss the importance of physical examinations, indications for tests, and tests to be included; and explain signs that indicate that the individual should seek professional help.

3. Explain the value of a home medicine chest, some items to be included, measures for safe storage of medications, and the use of over-the-counter medications.

Study Assignments

Pay careful attention to the following assignments. The chapter number may not be the same as the lesson number.

Textbook: Chapter 19, "Medical Care in America," pp. 482-492

Video: "Health Self-Care"

Key Terms

Watch for these terms and pay particular attention to what each one means, as you follow the textbook and video.

Generic name
Over-the-counter drugs (OTC)

Text Focus Points

Before you read the textbook assignment, review the following points to help focus your thoughts. After you complete the assignment, write out your responses to reinforce what you have learned.

1. Discuss current trends in health responsibility and the importance of being health-activated.

2. What are some of the characteristics and behaviors of the health-activated person?

3. Identify several of the body's "norms" and explain some of the factors that may cause them to vary.

4. Explain the need for a home medicine chest, some items to be included, and several measures for the safe storage of medications.

5. What is the value of regular physical examinations, and what are some of the tests that should be included? Explain when these tests should be considered.

6. Discuss factors that indicate the individual should seek professional medical help.

Experts Interviewed

In the video segment of this lesson, the following medical and health professionals share their expertise to help you understand the material presented.

Marvin Greenberg, R.Ph., Owner and Pharmacist in Charge, Greenberg's Drugs, Dallas, Texas

Elizabeth H. Gremore, R.N., M.S., C.H.E.S., Health Education Coordinator, McKinley Health Center, University of Illinois at Urbana-Champaign, Urbana, Illinois

Albert G. Mulley, Jr., M.D., M.P.P., Chief, General Internal Medicine, Massachusetts General Hospital, Boston, Massachusetts

Louis W. Sullivan, M.D., President, Morehouse School of Medicine, Atlanta, Georgia, Former Secretary, U.S. Department of Health and Human Services

Video Focus Points

The following questions are designed to help you get the most from the video segment of this lesson. Review them before you watch the video. After viewing the video segment, write responses to reinforce what you have learned.

1. Describe some of the problems that an individual can treat without seeking professional medical care. Include the signs and symptoms that indicate that professional care is needed.

2. What are the behaviors that indicate that a person is health-activated or proactive in maintaining good health?

3. Under what circumstances are over-the-counter medications useful? How does one choose a medication for a particular problem?

4. What are some of the important goals and concerns for the health of the American people in the future?

Individual Health Plan

This portion of the lesson is designed to enable you to apply the information you have learned to your own life situation and improve the quality of your life. You should do any exercise assigned, complete the journal portion of the plan, then put this portion of the health plan into practice in your life.

> In your journal, list the characteristics about yourself that you consider to be health-activated or non health-activated. Based on this, develop a written plan for yourself that will help you become more health-activated. If you are not keeping up with recommended physical examinations, do so.

Enrichment Opportunities

These suggestions guide you if you want more information on this lesson, want to explore new ideas, or if your instructor requires it. If you are doing this section as a course requirement, consult with your instructor for specific guidelines or directions.

1. Take an inventory of the over-the-counter (OTC) drugs in your home. Check the expiration dates and discard any that are out of date. Do the same for any prescription drugs you have.

2. In a visit to your pharmacy, read the labels of several OTC drugs meant for the same condition. Do you find similarities? Differences? Note the number of ingredients and the cost of each.

3. As you see advertisements for health care products, look for signs of quackery, misrepresentation, "stretching the truth."

Practice Test

After reading the assignment and watching the video, you should be able to answer the Practice Test questions. Tests also include essay questions that are similar to the Text Focus Points, the Video Focus Points, and the Objectives. When you have completed the Practice Test questions, turn to the Answer Key to score your answers.

1. Being self-activated about one's health is important because it
   A. helps one choose the most appropriate alternative health care.
   B. increases awareness of money spent on treatment of minor ailments.
   C. enhances one's sense of control over one's body.
   D. eliminates the need for health professionals.

2. When health-activated individuals assume more responsibility for their overall health, their goals are NOT likely to include
   A. realizing when to seek professional care.
   B. eliminating the role of health professionals.
   C. knowing which health professional to consult.
   D. making the best use of medical advice and expertise.

3. Which of the following conditions usually suggests infection?
   A. Respiration deeper than normal
   B. Body temperature more than a few degrees above 98.6 F
   C. Pulse rate lower than 60 beats per minute
   D. Blood pressure higher than 140/90

4. Which of the following is NOT a good way to organize a medicine chest?
   A. Stocking medical supplies for all possible illnesses
   B. Marking all over-the-counter medications with the date purchased
   C Locking drugs away from children
   D. Using drugs before their expiration dates

5. During a physical examination, a doctor should take a patient's medical history in order to
   A. spot potentially adverse conditions.
   B. determine current health status.
   C. assess past and present health status.
   D. identify dental abnormalities.

6. Which of the following recurring symptoms is LEAST likely to indicate need for medical help?
   A. Cold sweat combined with light-headedness
   B. Shortness of breath at rest
   C. Shortness of breath because of exertion
   D. Severe pain

7. The individual usually does NOT need to see a physician for
   A. abdominal pains.
   B. common colds.
   C. temperatures of 104 degrees F.
   D. earaches.

8. Behaviors that indicate a person is health-activated and being proactive in health include all the following EXCEPT
   A. exercising regularly.
   B. eating a healthy diet.
   C. refraining from seeing a physician except for emergencies.
   D. doing self-assessments of one's health.

9. Over-the-counter medications are useful to
   A. alleviate symptoms of minor ailments.
   B. eliminate infections.
   C. prevent colds and flu.
   D. cure many diseases.

10. Goals for improving the health of the people of the U.S. include all the following EXCEPT
    A. decreasing violence.
    B. strengthening the family.
    C. increasing dependence on physicians.
    D. improving nutrition.

11. Medicines that may be purchased without a prescription are called
    _____.

12. In a healthy adult at rest, the normal heart rate is _____ beats per minute.

13. A woman with a family history of breast cancer should have an annual _____.

14. A person who is proactive and takes responsibility for individual health is termed _____.

True or False

15. The current trend is toward depending more on physicians to maintain our health.

16. Seeking a second opinion in the case of serious illness is frequently a good idea.

17. Though medicines may interact with each other, foods and drinks rarely interact with drugs.

18. Any person experiencing abnormal symptoms should seek a medical opinion.

19. It is usually safe for individuals to treat their colds and minor wounds by themselves.

20. In spite of advertising claims, many over-the-counter medications have similar ingredients.

Answer Key

These are the correct answers with reference to the Learning Objectives, and to the source of the information: the Textbook Focus Points, Levy, *et al. Life and Health,* and the Video Focus Points. Page numbers are also given for the Textbook Focus Points. "KT" indicates questions with Key Terms defined.

Question	Answer	Learning Objective	Textbook Focus Point (page no.)	Video Focus Point
1.	C	23.1	1 (p. 483)	
2.	B	23.1	2 (p. 484)	
3.	B	23.2	3 (pp. 487-489)	
4	A	23.3	4 (p. 489)	
5	C	23.2	5 (p. 490)	
6	C	23.2	6 (p. 492)	
7	B	23.2		1
8	C	23.1		2
9	A	23.3		3
10	C	23.1		4
11.	over-the-counter drugs (OTC)	23.1	2 (p. 486)	KT
12.	60 to 90	23.2	3 (p. 488)	
13.	mammogram	23.2	5 (p. 491)	
14.	health-activated	23.1		2
15.	F	23.1	1 (p. 483)	
16.	T	23.1	2 (p. 485)	
17.	F	23.3	4 (p. 490)	
18.	T	23.2	6 (p. 491)	
19.	T	23.2		1
20.	T	23.3		3

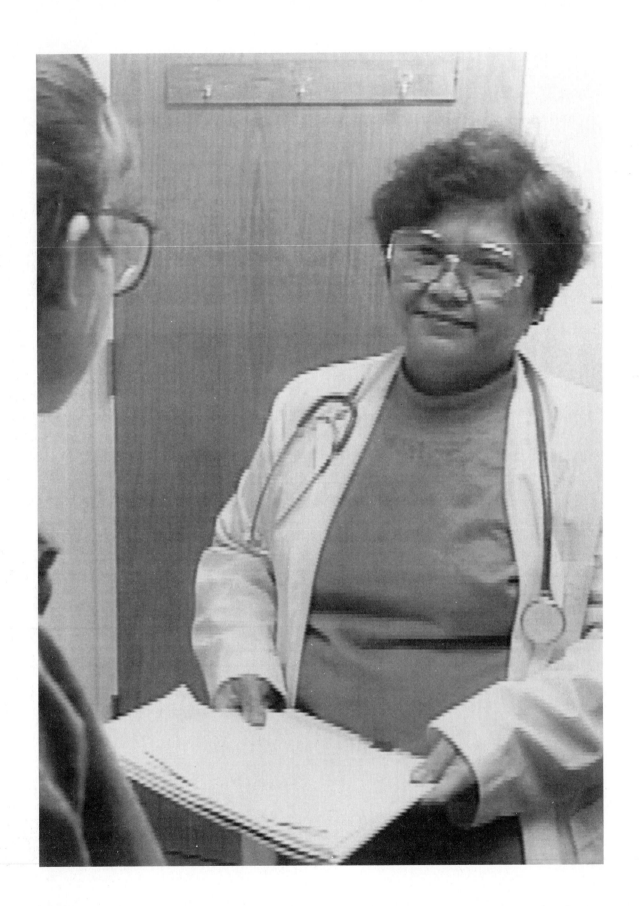

Lesson 24

Health Care Delivery Systems

The practice of medicine in its broadest sense includes the whole relationship of the physician with his patient. Good practice presupposes an understanding of modern medicine, but it is obvious that sound professional training should include a much broader equipment.

Dr. Francis Peabody, *JAMA;* 1927
(Journal of the American Medical Association)

Overview

If there is any question about our interest and concern about health care delivery systems, just read a newspaper, listen to a television newscast, or listen to a political speech. The whole country seems preoccupied with the large issue of health care. Unfortunately, we frequently don't understand the relationships that we as individuals have with this huge issue. We ask ourselves: "How do we fit in? What should we do? What can we really do?" Though we may feel there are no answers to all this, there really are some things that we as individuals can do.

Clearly, the most important thing that we can do is make lifestyle decisions that insure we keep ourselves as healthy as possible. Second, we can educate ourselves so that we are wise patients who take an active role in our recovery if we become ill. We should carefully choose our health care providers so we work with them as a team to maintain our health. We should be clear and reasonable about our health needs and expectations and intelligently evaluate the care we receive. We must **not** be passive consumers of health care who give up our rights when we enter the health care delivery system. Third, we must do what we can to help control the costs of health care. This involves using all the things we have learned to be health-activated and health-conscious.

If each of us from the single individual to the largest institution truly becomes involved in doing our part, the health care delivery system and problems in this country will surely "take a turn for the better."

Learning Objectives

Goal: You should be able to describe current trends in health care providers and delivery systems, compare and contrast various types of health insurance, and discuss ways you can control health care costs.

Objectives: Upon completion of this lesson, you should be able to:

1. Describe recent trends in health care providers, discuss several factors in selecting, communicating with, and assessing health care professionals and institutions, and describe several alternative types of health care.

2. Compare and contrast the various types of health insurance, including the HMO as an alternative.

3. Identify reasons for rising health care costs, and discuss the role of the individual in helping to control these costs.

Study Assignments

Pay careful attention to the following assignments. The chapter number may not be the same as the lesson number.

Textbook: Chapter 19, "Medical Care in America," pp. 493-507

Video: "Health Care Delivery Systems"

Key Terms

Watch for these terms and pay particular attention to what each one means, as you follow the textbook and video.

JCAH accreditation

"Patient's bill of rights"

Basic health insurance

Major medical insurance

Disability insurance

Group policies

Individual policies

Medicare

Medicaid

Health maintenance organization (HMO)

HMO group practice

Text Focus Points

Before you read the textbook assignment, review the following points to help focus your thoughts. After you complete the assignment, write out your responses to reinforce what you have learned.

1. Describe recent trends in health care providers in the United States.

2. Identify and discuss several factors in selecting, assessing, and communicating with a health care professional.

3. What role do hospitals, medicenters, and clinics play in the health care system? What are some of the issues to consider in assessing and dealing with health care institutions? Include discussion of the "patient's bill of rights."

4. What is meant by complementary approaches to health care? Identify and describe several alternative approaches to health care and treatment.

5. Compare and contrast the various types of health insurance, including government-funded programs. What is the most urgent health policy issue today?

6. What are the advantages and disadvantages of HMOs compared with traditional health care delivery systems?

7. Identify some of the reasons for rising health care costs and discuss ways in which individuals can help control the high costs of health care.

Expert Interviewed

In the video segment of this lesson, the following medical professional shares her expertise to help you understand the material presented.

Mary Ellen Hernandez Bluntzer, M.D., Internal Medicine, Family Systems Medicine, Dallas, Texas

Video Focus Points

The following questions are designed to help you get the most from the video segment of this lesson. Review them before you watch the video. After viewing the video segment, write responses to reinforce what you have learned.

1. Why is it so important to be an informed patient and to be actively involved in one's own health care?

2. Describe some guidelines that should be used when choosing and evaluating a health care provider.

3. What are the important factors in maintaining good communications between patient and physician? Include a discussion of the patient's rights.

Individual Health Plan

This portion of the lesson is designed to enable you to apply the information you have learned to your own life situation and improve the quality of your life. You should do any exercise assigned, complete the journal portion of the plan, then put this portion of the health plan into practice in your life.

In your journal, list your own resources for health care: physician, dentist, clinic, hospital insurance, etc. Describe the ways you utilize these services. Are you health-activated and health-conscious? If there are ways in which you could improve, develop a plan for doing this.

Enrichment Opportunities

These suggestions guide you if you want more information on this lesson, want to explore new ideas, or if your instructor requires it. If you are doing this section as a course requirement, consult with your instructor for specific guidelines or directions.

1. Compare and contrast health insurance plans, coverage, and cost of several different companies. Include Medicare and Medicaid. What were your findings?

2. Interview some physicians, dentists, and acquaintances of yours and find out their expectations of the health professional/patient relationship.

Practice Test

After reading the assignment and watching the video, you should be able to answer the Practice Test questions. Tests also include essay questions that are similar to the Text Focus Points, the Video Focus Points, and the Objectives. When you have completed the Practice Test questions, turn to the Answer Key to score your answers.

1. Which of the following is NOT an accurate portrayal of trends impacting people who seek health care?
   A. Fewer physicians in general practice
   B. Fewer physicians in rural areas
   C. More physicians in the inner city
   D. More dentists who are specializing

2. The LEAST important factor to consider when selecting a health professional is the professional's
   A. income.
   B. qualifications.
   C. philosophy of care.
   D. demeanor.

3. Hospitals play a crucial role in the health care system in all of the following ways EXCEPT by providing
   A. wide range of medical care.
   B. high-tech diagnostic equipment.
   C. high-risk patients access to medicenters and clinics.
   D. advanced life-support systems.

4. What is meant by complementary approaches to health care?
   A. Picturing positive mental images in order to improve some medical conditions
   B. Using nonconventional therapies in partnership with conventional medicine
   C. Funding medical research by both the government and the pharmaceutical industry
   D. Investing in nonconventional therapies for short-term treatments

5. Which hospitalization insurance program is funded by contributions to Social Security?
   A. Major medical insurance
   B. Disability insurance
   C. Medicaid
   D. Medicare

6. One advantage HMOs have over traditional health care is that HMOs
   A. encourage patients to "think preventively."
   B. offer more services.
   C. encourage hospitals to give more care.
   D. offer patients a wider choice of physicians.

7. Which of the following is NOT a reason for soaring health care costs?
   A. Doctor and hospital fees
   B. Expensive technology
   C. Increased use of medical services
   D. Laws to discourage competition among hospitals

8. A second opinion is usually NOT needed when the
    A. individual and physician agree about treatment.
    B. need for major surgery is indicated.
    C. individual questions the treatment.
    D. diagnosis is unclear.

9. Steps in choosing a physician do NOT include
    A. checking with the local medical society.
    B. interviewing several physicians.
    C. looking in the yellow pages of the phone book.
    D. considering the environment in the office.

10. The most important aspect in making an accurate diagnosis is the
    A. electrocardiogram.
    B. patient's history.
    C. blood tests.
    D. physical exam.

11. The list of rights the American Hospital Association has issued for hospital patients is called _____.

12. An individual who cannot work because of a knee injury is paid benefits by _____ insurance.

True or False
13. The *Directory of Medical Specialists,* published by the American Medical Association, is a good source of information about physicians.

14. In some cases, acupuncture or hypnosis have been as effective as painkillers for relieving pain.

15. In general, people should not choose a nonconventional approach to health care over a conventional approach.

16. Major medical insurance is designed to protect people from the high cost of catastrophic types of illness or injury.

17. The patient who takes an active role in treatment usually has a better outcome.

18. The general office environment is of little importance in the choice of a physician.

19. If either the physician or the patient questions the diagnosis or treatment plan, a second opinion should be sought.

20. Though many rights are maintained, the right to privacy must be given up when seeking medical treatment.

Answer Key

These are the correct answers with reference to the Learning Objectives, and to the source of the information: the Textbook Focus Points, Levy, *et al. Life and Health,* and the Video Focus Points. Page numbers are also given for the Textbook Focus Points. "KT" indicates questions with Key Terms defined.

Question	Answer	Learning Objective	Textbook Focus Point (page no.)	Video Focus Point
1.	C	24.1	1 (p. 494)	
2.	A	24.1	2 (pp. 495-496)	
3.	C	24.1	3 (p. 497)	
4.	B	24.1	4 (p. 499)	
5.	D	24.2	5 (p. 503)	KT
6.	A	24.2	6 (p. 505)	
7.	D	24.3	7 (p. 501)	
8.	A	24.1		1
9.	C	24.1		2
10.	B	24.1		3
11.	"patient's bill of rights"	24.1	3 (p. 498)	KT
12.	disability	24.2	5 (p. 503)	KT
13.	T	24.1	2 (p. 495)	
14.	T	24.1	4 (p. 499)	
15.	T	24.1	4 (p. 501)	
16.	T	24.2	5 (p. 503)	KT
17.	T	24.1		1
18.	F	24.1		2
19.	T	24.1		3
20.	F	24.1		3

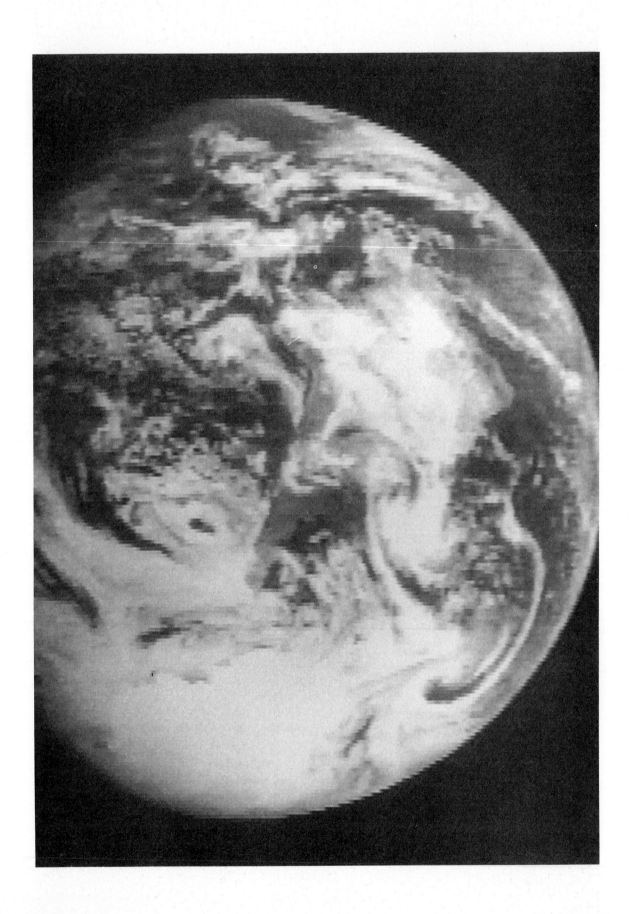

Lesson 25

Environmental Health

The whole point is we're on a road now that is leading to extinction. What we're doing now to the planet and the ways we do it are not sustainable . . . If we remember that our health and the health of the planet are synonymous, inseparable, then we'll start behaving differently toward the planet because we want health.

Hal Flanders

Overview

The technological revolution of the 20th century has at one time been a boon and a curse to the planet and its people. On the one hand, it has brought advances and wonders beyond belief. On the other, it seems to be dooming the planet to an early death.

As we consider the relationship of the environment and our health, we must realize that these two are inextricably intertwined. The health of the planet is our health and our health is the health of the planet. Each affects the other in more ways than we might imagine. All of the issues of advancing technology and their environmental impact are trade-offs. We cannot nor should we do without the health benefits that technology offers us. However, we cannot ignore the fact that the health of our planet is deteriorating rapidly and having damaging effects on our health. We cannot continue to use up our natural resources and pollute our air and water as though these are infinite. They are finite, and if they are depleted or polluted beyond use, we will become extinct as other species of the earth already have. Of all the dilemmas facing us, this is perhaps the most critical to our future. We can no longer hang on to the belief that technology will solve these problems. We must act individually to solve the simpler problems and then cooperatively develop solutions to the complex ones if our planet and its peoples are to survive and thrive.

Learning Objectives

Goal: You should be able to discuss the cyclical nature of the impact of the environment on the individual's health and the impact of the individual on the health of the environment, the extent to which pollution affects the health of the population, various environmental health problems, and important individual and cooperative action necessary to help solve these.

Objectives: Upon completion of this lesson, you should be able to:

1. Explain the extent to which pollution affects the world, discuss the way in which each type of pollution affects the health of the individual, and describe measures for dealing with the various types of pollution.

2. Discuss the environmental health problems related to the threat to the ozone layer, global warming, and deforestation.

3. Discuss the problems of the world's food supply and the effect of overpopulation on environmental problems.

4. Explain the relationship of energy use and the environment, including alternative forms of energy and the issues of nuclear power.

5. Describe important individual and cooperative actions necessary to help solve environmental health problems.

Study Assignments

Pay careful attention to the following assignments. The chapter number may not be the same as the lesson number.

Textbook: Chapter 20, "Health and the Environment," pp. 508-530

Video: "Environmental Health"

Key Terms

Watch for these terms and pay particular attention to what each one means, as you follow the textbook and video.

Pollution	Superfund
Carcinogens	Ozone layer
Ozone	Chlorofluorocarbons
Carrying capacity	Greenhouse effect
Chlorinated hydrocarbons	Deforestation
Polychlorinated biphenyls (PCBs)	Famine
Mercury	Methane
Acid rain	Hydroelectric power
Eutrophication	Chernobyl
Thermal pollution	Biodegradation
Landfill	

Text Focus Points

Before you read the textbook assignment, review the following points to help focus your thoughts. After you complete the assignment, write out your responses to reinforce what you have learned.

1. What is pollution and what does it affect? How is technology involved?

2. Identify various types of air pollution and discuss the ways that each affects the health of the individual. What was the purpose of the Clean Air Act of 1970?

3. How important is our regional water supply? Identify various types of water pollution and discuss the ways that each affects the health of the individual. What is being done to improve water quality?

4. How much hazardous waste is produced every year in the United States? Describe the Love Canal incident. Describe Superfund and other methods of dealing with hazardous waste. Identify household hazardous waste products and describe methods for dealing with nonhazardous household waste.

5. Describe how the earth's ozone layer, temperature, forests, and land are interconnected. Describe how they are being damaged and what consequences the damage has on us and the world. Identify ways in which we can reverse this trend.

6. Explain the effect of increased energy efficiency on environmental problems. Describe several alternative sources of energy, including the pros and cons of nuclear power.

7. How is cooperative action important in dealing with environmental problems?

8. Describe ways in which individuals can help solve environmental problems.

Experts Interviewed

In the video segment of this lesson, the following health professionals share their expertise to help you understand the material presented.

Andres E. Garcia-Rivera, M.S., Director, Environmental Health, Cornell University, Ithaca, New York

Amy Martin, Environmental Science Writer, Dallas, Texas

Video Focus Points

The following questions are designed to help you get the most from the video segment of this lesson. Review them before you watch the video. After viewing the video segment, write responses to reinforce what you have learned.

1. Explain the cyclical process of the impact that individuals have on the environment and the environment has on the individual.

2. Why is it important to be involved in individual and cooperative action to protect the health of the environment and in turn our own health?

3. What are some of the things that individuals can do every day to improve the health of the environment and themselves?

Individual Health Plan

This portion of the lesson is designed to enable you to apply the information you have learned to your own life situation and improve the quality of your life. You should do any exercise assigned, complete the journal portion of the plan, then put this portion of the health plan into practice in your life.

Complete the self-assessment, "How Knowledgeable Are You About the Environment?" on pages 512-513 of your text. In your journal, list any health problems you have that could be caused or affected by environmental factors. List and discuss actions you take that either add to or detract from the health of the environment. On the basis of these factors, develop a plan to do your part in improving the health of the planet and in turn your own health.

Enrichment Opportunity

This suggestion guides you if you want more information on this lesson, want to explore new ideas, or if your instructor requires it. If you are doing this section as a course requirement, consult with your instructor for specific guidelines or directions.

Interview local representatives of private and government environmental protection agencies and find out what major environmental problems exist in your area, what is being done to improve these, and what role you might play in the solution.

Practice Test

After reading the assignment and watching the video, you should be able to answer the Practice Test questions. Tests also include essay questions that are similar to the Text Focus Points, the Video Focus Points, and the Objectives. When you have completed the Practice Test questions, turn to the Answer Key to score your answers.

1. On which of the following has pollution had the greatest effect?
   A. Economics and social planning
   B. People's physical health
   C. Values and desires
   D. Technological innovations

2. Which of the following substances is associated with an increased risk of developing lung and intestinal cancer?
   A. Asbestos
   B. Carbon monoxide
   C. PCBs
   D. Mercury

3. What chemicals in the water supply have been linked to reproductive disorders, kidney damage, and liver ailments?
   A. Polychlorinated biphenyls (PCBs)
   B. Chlorinated hydrocarbons
   C. Particulate matter
   D. Sulfur oxides

4. Every year the United States produces about how much hazardous waste per person?
   A. 1 ton
   B. 1,000 pounds
   C. 500 pounds
   D. 250 pounds

5. All of the following are risks to human health caused by depletion of the earth's ozone layer EXCEPT
   A. cardiovascular disorders.
   B. skin cancer.
   C. cataracts.
   D. decreased resistance to viral disease.

6. A viable alternative to fossil fuels in the future is LEAST likely to be
   A. solar power.
   B. hydroelectric power.
   C. wind power.
   D. human power.

7. Efforts that each individual can make to help protect the environment are LEAST likely to include
   A. driving individual cars.
   B. using more biodegradable materials.
   C. recycling.
   D. actively working on environmental issues.

8. The relationship of humans to the other species on the planet can be described as
   A. advanced.
   B. separate.
   C. interrelated.
   D. independent.

9. Solving environmental health problems does NOT include more
   A. political policy.
   B. individual action.
   C. cooperative efforts.
   D. technological development.

10. A sign of the air quality in an area is the
    A. velocity of the wind.
    B. growth of lichens.
    C. amount of acid rain.
    D. density of the trees.

11. Undesirable substances and forms of energy that have destructive effects on the physical environment are known as _____.

12. A group of dangerous chemicals used in the manufacture of electrical equipment is _____.

13. If the world's food supplies are not protected, extreme shortages of food may result and cause widespread _____.

14. The relationship between the health of the individual and the health of the environment is _____.

True or False
15. Landfills designed to hold nonhazardous waste are constantly increasing in number.

16. If the United States and a few of the other large countries solved their environmental problems, the environmental problems of the world would be solved.

17. The relationship between the health of the environment and the health of the individual is a cyclical one.

18. A key to solving community, environmental problems is through cooperative action.

19. There are few areas in the United States that have very low amounts of air pollution.

20. Eating higher on the food chain, with more processed and prepackaged foods, will increase individual health and the health of the environment.

Answer Key

These are the correct answers with reference to the Learning Objectives, and to the source of the information: the Textbook Focus Points, Levy, *et al. Life and Health,* and the Video Focus Points. Page numbers are also given for the Textbook Focus Points. "KT" indicates questions with Key Terms defined.

Question	Answer	Learning Objective	Textbook Focus Point (page no.)	Video Focus Point
1.	B	25.1	1 (p. 509)	
2.	A	25.1	2 (p. 514)	
3.	A	25.1	3 (p. 515)	
4.	A	25.1	4 (p. 517)	
5.	A	25.2	5 (p. 520)	
6.	D	25.4	6 (p. 523)	
7.	A	25.5	8 (pp. 526-528)	
8.	C	25.1		1
9.	D	25.5		2
10.	B	25.5		2
11.	pollution or pollutants	25.1	1 (p. 509	KT
12.	PCBs	25.1	3 (p. 515	KT
13.	famine	25.3	5 (p. 522)	KT
14.	cyclical or interrelated	25.1		1
15.	F	25.1	4 (p. 519)	
16.	F	25.5	7 (p. 525)	
17.	T	25.1		1
18.	T	25.5		2
19.	T	25.5		2
20.	F	25.5		3

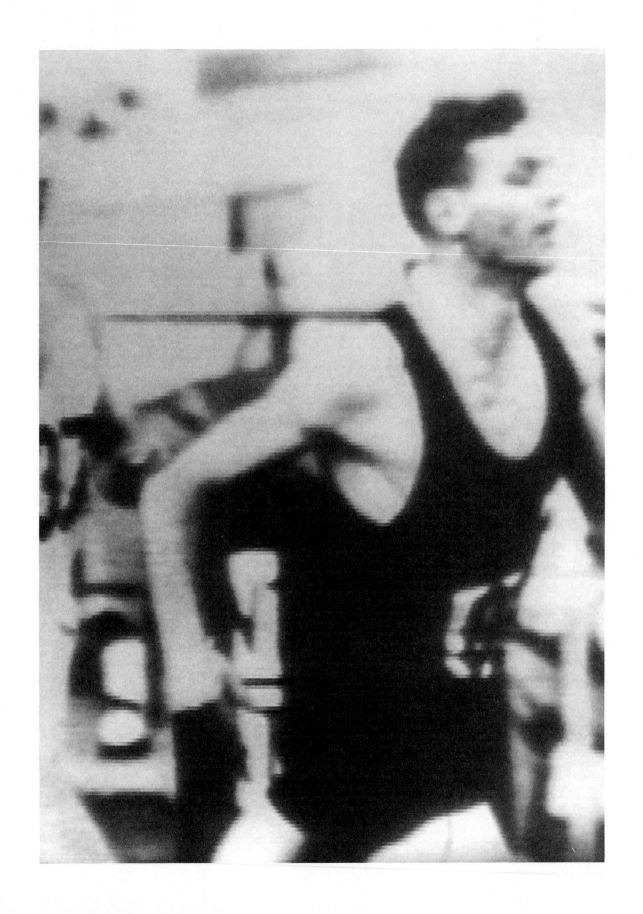

Lesson 26

A Celebration of Health

I truly believe that every human being consists of a physical, an emotional, an intellectual, and a spiritual quadrant . . . which work together in total harmony and wholeness . . . It is only if we have learned to accept our physicalness, if we love and accept our natural emotions without being handicapped by them, without being belittled when we cry, when we express natural anger, when we are jealous in order to emulate someone else's talents, gifts, or behavior. Then we will be able to understand that we have only two natural fears, one of falling and one of loud noises. All other fears have been given to us by grown-ups who projected their own fears onto us, and have passed them from generation to generation.

Most important of all, we must learn to love and to be loved unconditionally. Most of us have been raised as prostitutes. I will love you 'if.' And this word 'if' has ruined and destroyed more lives than anything else on this planet earth. It prostitutes us, it makes us feel we can buy love with good behavior or good grades. We will never develop a sense of self-love and self-reward. If we were not able to accommodate the grown-ups, we were punished, rather than being taught by consistent loving discipline. As our teachers taught, if you had been raised with unconditional love and discipline, you will never be afraid of the windstorms of life. You would have no fear, no guilt, and no anxieties, the only enemies of men. Should you shield the canyon from the windstorms, you would never see the beauty of their carvings.

Elisabeth Kübler-Ross, M.D., *On Life After Death*

A Celebration of Health

Overview

We have shared a long journey, you and I, over the miles, through lives, experiences, and learning. Soon we will part, each to continue our own life. Before we part, think back to the beginning. Remember we talked about the five dimensions of health: physical, emotional, intellectual, social, and spiritual. How many times we have seen these in people's lives? How many times we have heard them talk of these? Even more important we have talked about our lifestyle decisions and choices, that either increase the quality of our health or detract from it. As you think back, think of all the different people you have met, some very like yourself, some very different. If you saw yourself in some of the people and situations, was it with celebration or was it with pain?

We have a few more people to meet before we part. All the people you have met have been special in their own way. The people you will now meet you may or may not recognize. Each has made lifestyle decisions to expand one of the dimensions of their health beyond that which most of us achieve. Each started their personal journey to health in much the same way as you and I, but somewhere along the way, they made some incredible decisions in their own lifestyle. Their life now is, as yours and mine, a reflection of these decisions and their outcomes. As you meet them, think of your own life and health. What decisions have you made? What lifestyle choices and decisions will you make? Your future and your health are up to you. My hope is that the future will find you **living with health!**

Learning Objectives

Goal: You should be able to apply the concept of health in the five dimensions; physical, emotional, intellectual, social, and spiritual to your own life and describe aspects of your own lifestyle that support your health and well-being in the five dimensions.

Objectives: Upon completion of this lesson, you should be able to:

1. Explain the aspects of your own lifestyle that improve the physical dimension of your health.

---

2. Discuss the aspects of your own lifestyle that develop the emotional dimension of your health.

3. Analyze the aspects of your own lifestyle that expand the intellectual dimension of your health.

4. Discuss the aspects of your own lifestyle that sustain the social dimension of your health.

5. Describe the aspects of your own lifestyle that deepen the spiritual dimension of your health.

Study Assignments

Pay careful attention to the following assignments. The chapter number may not be the same as the lesson number.

Textbook: Review Chapter 1, and others that you feel you need.

Video: "A Celebration of Health"

Key Terms

There are no new terms in this lesson.

Textbook and Video Focus Points

The following questions are designed to help you get the most from the textbook review assignment and the video segment of this lesson. Review them before you watch the video. After reviewing the textbook chapters and viewing the video segment, write responses to reinforce what you have learned.

1. What are the changes in your own physical health lifestyle that support your health? Examine diet, exercise, rest, alcohol, drug and medication use, tobacco use, and other aspects that impact physical health. What are your future plans and goals?

---

2. How have you grown in your emotional health lifestyle choices? Examine your self-concept, self-esteem, coping abilities, relationships with others, stress management activities, alcohol and drug use, and other aspects that influence emotional health. What do you plan for the future?

3. How have you increased lifestyle behaviors in the intellectual dimension? Examine your study habits, learning activities, working patterns, choices in books, movies, and television, and any other activities that support your intellectual growth. What goals and plans do you have for the future?

4. What lifestyle decisions have you made to enhance the social dimension of your health? Examine leisure time activities, relationships with family and friends, community volunteer activities, and other aspects that influence the social portion of your well-being. What plans have you made for the future?

5. How do your behaviors, beliefs, and values support the spiritual dimension of your life? Examine the relationship of your behavior with your beliefs and values, your respect for others, valuing of the environment, and other aspects that develop the spiritual dimensions.

Experts Interviewed

In the video segment of this lesson, the following professionals share their expertise to help you understand the material presented.

Liz Carpenter, Author, Lecturer, and Journalist, Austin, Texas

Sara Hickman, Musician, Artist, and Humanitarian, Dallas, Texas

Barbara Jordan, LL.D., Lyndon B. Johnson Centennial Chair in National Policy, The Lyndon B. Johnson School of Public Affairs, The University of Texas, Austin, Texas

Peter G. Snell, Ph.D., Olympic Gold Medalist - 800 m - 1960, Olympic Gold Medalist - 800 m - 1964, Olympic Gold Medalist - 1500 m - 1964, Assistant Professor of Medicine and Physiology, The University of Texas Southwestern Medical Center, Dallas, Texas

Julian D. Pinkham, M.S., M.S.W., Member, Yakima Indian Nation, Toppenish, Washington

Individual Health Plan

This portion of the lesson is designed to enable you to apply the information you have learned to your own life situation and improve the quality of your life. You should do any exercise assigned, complete the journal portion of the plan, then put this portion of the health plan into practice in your life.

> After reviewing your health, lifestyle status, and goals at the beginning and throughout the course, in your journal, write an evaluation of the present status of your health and lifestyle. Has your health changed or improved in any way? What progress have you made toward goals you have set? Have you changed any of your goals and plans? Update your lifestyle plan for the immediate future and for your long-term health goals.

Enrichment Opportunities

These suggestions guide you if you want more information on this lesson, want to explore new ideas, or if your instructor requires it. If you are doing this section as a course requirement, consult with your instructor for specific guidelines or directions.

> Select someone you know that you think exemplifies a lifestyle that is well-balanced among the five dimensions. Talk with that person and find out what lifestyle choices, decisions, and even trade-offs have been necessary to achieve this balance.

Practice Test

There are no new objective test items in this lesson. Your Individual Health Plan serves as your review essay questions.